BABY SLEEP TRAINING:

GET YOUR BABY TO SLEEP THROUGH THE NIGHT IN 4 EASY-TO-FOLLOW STEPS

Give Your Baby and Yourself the Gift of A Good Night's Sleep Without Crying It Out

Grace Stockholm

© Copyright 2019 - All rights reserved.

The content contained within this book may not be reproduced, duplicated or transmitted without direct written permission from the author or the publisher.

Under no circumstances will any blame or legal responsibility be held against the publisher, or author, for any damages, reparation, or monetary loss due to the information contained within this book, either directly or indirectly.

Legal Notice:

This book is copyright protected. It is only for personal use. You cannot amend, distribute, sell, use, quote or paraphrase any part, or the content within this book, without the consent of the author or publisher.

Disclaimer Notice:

Please note the information contained within this document is for educational and entertainment purposes only. All effort has been executed to present accurate, up to date, reliable, complete information. No warranties of any kind are declared or implied. Readers acknowledge that the author is not engaged in the rendering of legal, financial, medical or professional advice. The content within this book has been derived from various sources. Please consult a licensed professional before attempting any techniques outlined in this book.

By reading this document, the reader agrees that under no circumstances is the author responsible for any losses, direct or indirect, that are incurred as a result of the use of information contained within this document, including, but not limited to, errors, omissions, or inaccuracies.

TABLE OF CONTENTS

INTRODUCTION 8

CHAPTER 1: The Factors of Healthy Sleeping 15

   Healthy Sleep Factors 15

   How Much Sleep Does Your Baby Need? 18

      0 to 3 Months 18

      3 to 5 Months 19

      5 to 8 Months 19

      8 to 15 Months 20

      16 to 36 Months 20

   What Does Healthy Sleep Look Like? 20

   Understanding Sleep Problems 21

      Common Sleep Disorders 21

   Understand Your Child's Sleeping Cues and Patterns 22

   Key Points to Remember 23

CHAPTER 2: The Importance of Healthy Sleeping 24

   Effects of Healthy Sleep 24

      0 to 3 Months 24

      3 to 5 Months 25

- 5 to 8 Months 26
- 8 to 15 Months 28
- 16 to 36 Months 29

Do Not Forget About Yourself 29

Effects of Sleep Deprivation 30

- When You Are Sleep Deprived 31
- When Your Baby Is Sleep Deprived 32

Key Points to Remember 34

CHAPTER 3: Your Baby's First Months – What to Expect and How to Start Implementing Healthy Sleep Practices 35

What Is the Fourth Trimester? 35

- What Are Your Baby's Needs During the Fourth Trimester? 36

Introducing Routines Into Your Baby's Life 38

- Daytime Routine 39
- Nighttime Routine 39
- Your Baby's Crib Is More Important Than You Think 40
- "Sleeping When Your Baby Sleeps" Is Just an Idea 40

Key Points to Remember 41

CHAPTER 4: The Importance of Answering Your Baby's Cry – Is There a No-Cry Method? 42

Is There a No-Cry Method to Sleep Training? 42

- Benefits of the No-Tears Method 43
- Establishing a No-Tears Method Routine 43

The Cry-It-Out Method 45

> What to Know About the Cry-It-Out Method..................................46

> *Answering Your Baby's Cries* 49

>> Types of Cries 49

>> Tips for Understanding Your Baby's Cries 51

> *Key Point to Remember*..52

CHAPTER 5: There Is No One Baby, There Is No One Book..................53

> *Every Baby Is Different* 54

> *The Process Is a Gradual One* 54

> *Key Points to Remember* 55

CHAPTER 6: Let's Get Sleeping, But First Thing's First – Safety 57

> *Sudden Infant Death Syndrome (SIDS)* 59

>> Back-to-Sleep Approach 62

> *Safety With Co-Sleeping*...63

> *Other Safety Tips*..65

> *Key Points to Remember* 67

CHAPTER 7: The Importance of Your Baby's Day and Nighttime Routine 68

> *Benefits of Routines* 68

> *Daily Schedules*...70

>> Daytime and Nighttime Feedings 70

>> Nighttime Routine 71

>> Nap Routine 74

> *Breaking the Nurse to Sleep Habit of Your Newborn* 76

> *Key Points to Remember* 78

CHAPTER 8: Ready, Set, Sleep 79

Tips to Help You During the Sleep Training Process 79

Four Steps of the Sleep Process 82

- Step One: Befriend the Bed 82
- Step Two: Weaning From Touch 83
- Step Three: Attendance Test 83
- Step Four: Goodnight, Darling 84

Daytime Sleep 85
Night Feedings 85
Key Points to Remember 86

CHAPTER 9: Sleep Regression and Problem Solving 87

Sleep Regression: It Is Real 87

- 4-Month Sleep Regression 88
- 8- or 10-Month Sleep Regression 90
- 11- or 12-Month Sleep Regression 93
- 18-Month Sleep Regression 96
- 2-Year Sleep Regression 100

Consistency Is the Key 106
Key Points to Remember 107

CHAPTER 10: Baby Is Sleeping but Are You? 109

Sleeping Problems of a Young Mother 109

- Sleep Apnea 112
- Postpartum Depression (PPD) 113

Postpartum Psychosis (PPP) 115

General Anxiety of a Young Mother *115*

Postpartum Anxiety and Obsessive-Compulsive Disorder (PPA/OCD) 116

Solutions for You *117*

Key Points to Remember *119*

CHAPTER 11: Personal Note – Mom to Mom 120

CONCLUSION 124

BONUS SECTION: Guided Meditation for Parents - Putting Your Baby to Sleep 126

RESOURCES 140

INTRODUCTION

You are here because you feel that you have been awake forever. You are sleep deprived and all you want is one night of full, uninterrupted sleep. You might feel that this is your last hope to get more sleep than you are currently getting right now.

The fact is one of the biggest problems for mothers is they are so sleep deprived that they have trouble functioning. You may be well aware of some of the areas of your life where you lack the energy to focus. You might make more mistakes at work, forget to run errands, and in some instances, you may even forget to pay bills. You might lack focus when you are taking care of your baby or driving. A good night's sleep is just as important to you as it is to your baby. You need to function your best, so you can give your baby the best care. With a good night's sleep, you will feel less stressed and be more content. You will have more patience, which will allow you to help teach your baby what they need to learn to thrive.

As a mother, you want to ensure that your baby is developing the best way they can. You want your baby to thrive from the moment you find out that you are pregnant, and this feeling becomes stronger once you give birth and bring them home. However, to help your baby thrive, you need to ensure that they are getting an adequate amount of sleep they need for their age. Your baby will suffer from similar side effects as you do when they lack sleep. They will have trouble focusing, which can delay their learning. They will become overtired, which means they will gain more energy and you will continue to struggle to get them to sleep.

Most people think that sleep comes naturally. However, this does not mean you should not help your child gain the skills needed to sleep through the night. Think of it this way: breastfeeding is one of the most natural things for a mother. Yet, there are many mothers who need help when it comes to breastfeeding. Nurses are trained to help mothers understand the basics of breastfeeding and what to do when they run into a problem. Sleeping is no different.

Sleep training is a way that you can teach your child to fall asleep on their own. There is one major misconception that immediately comes to mind when a parent hears this term. Sleep training does not require you to leave your baby alone to cry until they give up because they feel that you will not come and take care of what they need. You always attend to your baby's needs when you are sleep training. It is a gradual process that can take weeks. In fact, it can take over a month for some parents. Sleep training is empowering because it allows you to bond with your baby. It helps your baby's confidence grow as they learn that you will take care of them and will always be there when they need you. You will give them the tools they need to learn new skills. Through the four-step process you learn about in this book, you will help your baby learn to self-soothe themselves to sleep. They will not need you to help soothe them, unless there are other factors in play, such as an illness, teething, or sleep regression.

For almost a full year, my first son and I were co-sleeping. It was as though the days and nights began to blur together at some point. By the time my son was nine-months old, I was the typical sleep-deprived mom. And, despite all my efforts with breastfeeding, adding in bottle feedings and solids, my son was in the lower 3rd percentile for weight for a baby his age. I had been putting off sleep training because I feared cutting back on those night time feedings and him falling further behind in the weight category. I was miserable though, and so was everyone else in the house, including my sweet little boy. Despite my reluctance, we began sleep training.

We struggled the first few nights. I had a lot of guilt; many moms do. I didn't want to hear him crying but also knew that I didn't want him to depend on external elements to be able to fall and stay asleep. There were many times during those first few nights and days I almost caved. But then we began to fall into a routine and there was a noticeable shift in my sweet boy. He was actually the calm, happy baby he was before. He was eating like a champ and not just snacking constantly. During the day, he was attentive and playful. And at night, he slept peacefully. Though I began sleep training because I was beyond exhausted, the process benefitted him far more than I had ever realized it would. Seeing how much he was progressing after a good night's sleep is what motivated me to continue with the process. After just 10 days, he was sleeping through the night.

The thought of him skipping his nighttime feedings made me anxious. I thought for sure he would drop in weight, but the complete opposite happened. Little did I know his sleep-deprived body was unable to use the food he was eating properly. When he began to sleep through the night, he began to gain weight, and in just a short time, he was above the 30th percentile. It is not an exaggeration when I say that this process has changed our lives for the better, starting first and foremost with our son. He is so much happier now. Even though we run into the expected sleep regression periods, I know he has learned the skills he needs to be able to fall back into a healthy sleep pattern

Baby number two arrived by the time my oldest son had just turned two. The toddler years are full of energy, at least for my son. I had all the intentions of ensuring our newborn would fall into proper sleep patterns early on. But, with a newborn and toddler running around, I needed to squeeze in additional sleep whenever I could. It didn't take long for me to fall into the co-sleeping patterns with my second son as I had with my first. My second son would cry all night long. He refused to sleep, and it wasn't just at night. During the day he wouldn't nap, even if we walked with him in the stroller, rocked with him in a chair, or drove around with him in the car seat. When it was time for him to sleep at night, no matter where it was or what we did, he just didn't sleep. It seemed like all he did was cry and scream, and so much of our attention was being given to the baby that our sweet toddler was missing out on the attention that he also needed.

When we decided to sleep train with our second son, I felt some reluctance again. I had to remind myself of the positive impact it had on my first son and so we began. Almost instantly there was a noticeable change. The process was no easier; I still held him when he cried and could only tolerate hearing him cry for a short period of time, but when he slept, there was a significant change. We started the sleep training process earlier with our second son, so we knew that getting him to sleep through the night was still a few months away as he still needed his nighttime feedings. But what a difference we saw in his temperament when he actually napped during the day (and he rarely took naps prior to starting sleep training). We had no idea how easy going, fun, and bright-eyed our second son was. He laughed and played and was such a tremendous joy to be around. I am so thankful that we helped him learn the skill of sleeping at such a young age and enabled him to start enjoying life.

With a good night's sleep, both you and your baby will thrive. Sleep helps you maintain focus, helps your baby's eating habits, developmental process, and ensures your baby is comfortable, happy, and healthy. This will help you feel the same way. Your little one will have the energy to learn new skills and you will have the patience to teach your baby. Most importantly, you will begin to truly enjoy parenthood and realize that you will make it through the difficult parts.

If you have older children, this sleep training process will provide you with the time and energy to function and care for all of them. Having a new baby in the home can be uncomfortable and tense for the existing kids in the house as it is. Having a fussy, sleepless baby may make you edgy and short-tempered, which will directly affect all of your children. You may find yourself trying to put your baby down for his naps all day long, leaving you with no time for your other children, not to mention for yourself. Having a well-rested baby will allow you to care and give your children what they need, especially in this hectic period of bringing a new baby home. You will have energy and time to invest in them, as well as yourself, your spouse, the household, and anything else that is important for you. After a good night's sleep, everything seems less intimidating and you will thrive as a mom.

Sleep training provides parents with tailored steps that will help ease your baby into healthy sleeping patterns. The process can be customized to suit you and your family's needs. Most importantly, this four-step sleep training process ensures that you maintain that strong bond and connection with your baby. Celebrities like Hillary Duff and Chrissy Teigen have used sleep training techniques to get their first-born babies to sleep better. But, with the tips and guidelines in this book, you don't have to be a celebrity to benefit from the process.

In this book, you will learn many details about sleep training, such as:

- How much sleep your baby really needs.
- How to recognize your baby's sleep cues and decode their different cries so you can better understand when they are tired, and when they need to be fed, changed, or are just bored.
- How to use a schedule that is flexible and right for you, so your baby can eat at relatively the same time each day while still not

going hungry.
- How to teach your baby to soothe themselves so that they can relax and fall asleep on their own.
- When and how to start sleep training and learn what to do in each step of the way.
- How to master the bedtime routine so it will go from being the most dreaded part of the day to the most enjoyable, quality time spent with your baby.

This book will outline how to teach your baby the skills they need to get a long night of quality sleep. Your baby is already equipped with a number of natural biological skills, but even these natural skills won't help them get along in the world. It is our responsibility as parents to nurture them and teach them life-skills and utilize those natural skills as they grow and become more independent. Sleep is a vital basic need of any creature. Being able to soothe yourself and independently enter into a calm, good sleep is such a valuable skill to give your growing baby.

Sleep, just as with any other life skill, needs to be taught, practiced, and acquired. Many natural survival mechanisms, such as breastfeeding, need additional support and training from time to time. Breastfeeding is the most natural skill both mom and baby already possess, yet many mothers and their babies struggle with the process. Lactation specialist and counseling sessions are attended so that mom and baby can easily improve upon this natural skill so that they remain healthy and happy. Sleep is no different. Babies will need to learn the steps for healthy sleep and you, the parent, can teach them.

Being a tired, sleep-deprived mom does not win you an award for "Mom of the Year." In fact, a good mom is one that is full of just as much energy as her children! The sleep training method described in this book is a process that has not only worked wonderfully for both of my boys but for friends, family members, and hundreds of parents around the world. And it can do wonders for you and your baby as well.

<u>Before we move along, it is important to stress:</u> If you have concerns or questions about your baby's health, you should always consult with a physician or other health care professional. Do not disregard, avoid, or delay obtaining medical or health-related advice from your baby's health care professional because of something you may have read in this book.

CHAPTER 1: The Factors of Healthy Sleeping

One of the first steps you need to take when it comes to healthy sleep for your baby is to understand the different factors that promote healthy sleep. Each stage of growth for your baby has different factors that enables them to sleep well. Understanding these factors and stages allows you to know what to expect and how to encourage healthy sleep patterns in accordance to their age. In addition to being able to identify how much sleep your baby needs, you will want to know what to look out for when it comes to sleep problems and sleep cues your baby will exhibit.

Healthy Sleep Factors

There are five fundamental elements that negate healthy sleep patterns in children:

1. **The duration of sleep**. Your baby will need a specific amount of sleep each day to help assist their growing brains. Newborns will sleep for much longer periods of time than a three- or four-month-old, as newborns sleep in accordance with their sleep needs. After three or four months, in addition to factoring the duration of sleep your baby will get, the biggest factor to consider will be parental practices. It is important to understand that your baby needs to sleep enough in order to be a happier, healthier, and more peaceful child. Interfering with your child's sleep needs will disrupt their natural sleep process and will almost always result in a fussy child that simply

needs to sleep more.

2. **Naptime**. Naps are essential for cognitive development and are what allows your baby to be able to retain and learn all the new information they are exposed to on a daily basis. Naps allow for the night sleep, day sleep, and wakefulness cycle to fall into a synchronized rhythm. Naps allow babies to balance out their day sleep and wakefulness patterns. For the first four months, your baby will nap a number of times during the day simply because their brains have not developed enough to distinguish between when they should be awake and alert and when they should be resting. After about four months, babies will begin to use their naps as a way to continue their nighttime sleep (which occurs with the morning nap) and to give their bodies time to restore itself (which occurs with the afternoon and/or the early evening nap). The length of the nap and the time your baby is napping will affect the quality of sleep they get through the day. Babies who nap for longer in the afternoon are getting more restorative sleep. Your baby will be more alert and attentive after an afternoon nap than they usually are after their morning nap.

3. **Sleep consolidation.** Sleep consolidation refers to the uninterrupted sleep your baby is able to get. Sleep arousal and sleep fragmentation can be common occurrences that keep very young babies alive. It is these arousals that jolt us awake when we have difficulty breathing. After six or seven months, sleep fragmentation and arousal can begin to harm your baby as they take away from the actual sleep duration. Your baby may have partial awakenings, where they may awaken temporarily and fall immediately back to sleep. They may also have full awakenings where they attempt to fall back asleep but are unsuccessful. When your baby is fully awake, they become

completely aware of their surroundings, and even if they do eventually fall back asleep, these awakening take away from their total sleep durations. This can result in an overly tired and fussy baby during waking hours. Sleep awakening and arousal can occur during the evening hours as well as throughout nap times. In the evening, these waking hours tend to have a bigger impact on your baby's sleep consolidation because your child may not have the necessary skills before six months of age to fall promptly back to sleep on their own.

4. **Sleep schedule**. Sleep should be treated the same way as feeding your baby. You would never deprive your hungry baby of food when they cry for it just as you should never keep your baby awake when they are giving you clear signals they are tired. Up until six weeks old, they will sleep frequently but typically for short periods of time. Often the longest they will sleep is three hours. After the six-week mark, babies will begin to sleep longer in the evening, many up to five hours straight. Once your baby is around three months old, they will begin to have more regular daytime sleep patterns. Developing an effective sleep schedule is often a set of trial and error, and many parents try to create their child's sleep schedule in accordance with the parent's lifestyles. This is often not ideal for the baby. Many babies at a young age benefit more from an early bedtime than a later one. Parents tend to keep their babies up at night because they fear an earlier bedtime will result in an earlier waking time. This is often quite the opposite. For many babies, an earlier bedtime allows them to sleep the longer hours they need so they are more alert and active during the day.

5. **The regularity of sleep.** You should aim to put your baby to sleep when you first see signs of drowsiness. As you become

more aware of these sleepy signs your child gives, you will be able to know when to expect them. This will help you put your baby to bed at the same time every night, which will result in them getting the right amount of sleep. When you are about to begin sleep training with your baby, one of the first things you want to establish is a consistent bedtime and daytime sleep times. As your baby grows older, the times may need to be adjusted, either moved up or moved back, and for naps to be eliminated completely. What is important is to always establish a set time when sleep will occur.

When each of these elements of sleep is balanced appropriately, children are able to learn healthy sleep patterns. Each of these elements work together with one another and are not separate factors that stand alone. As your baby grows, these factors remain, though the timing, length, and implementation of them will vary. Let's take a look at how each of these factors comes into play for your growing baby.

How Much Sleep Does Your Baby Need?

The amount of sleep your baby needs as they grow will decrease with time. Sleep will change frequently as they begin to adjust to their new outside world. Knowing how much sleep they require and when to expect changes in their sleeping patterns will allow you to better create a sleep training plan that ensures your baby gets optimal sleep.

0 to 3 Months

From when a baby is born until three months, your baby should get about 15 to 17 hours of sleep during a 24-hour period. They will take several naps during the 24 hours but not many will be longer than two to three hours. Naps at this time are fairly irregular as your baby simply follows their own natural rhythm for sleep. When they are tired, they will sleep. You can expect nighttime sleep to follow the same patterns as daytime sleep. Your baby will wake up throughout the night for their feedings and diaper changes. One reason they tend to sleep for a few hours and then wake up for an hour or a little less is that they have no clear idea of the difference between night and day. You might start to notice that they are awake for longer periods of time closer to their third month.

3 to 5 Months

At three to five months, babies should get 15 hours of sleep during the 24-hour period. They will have a morning nap that lasts one and a half to two hours, a midday nap that lasts two to two and a half hours, and an afternoon nap that lasts about one hour. During the nighttime, they will sleep about nine and a half to 10 ½ hours, but this is often not uninterrupted sleep. They should have about three feedings during the night, and often wake every three or four hours.

5 to 8 Months

Between five and eight months of age, your baby should sleep 14 ½ hours in a 24-hour period. Their morning nap will be about one to one and a half hours, midday nap will be two to two and a half hours, and an afternoon nap will be a half an hour to one hour in length. They should sleep about nine and a half to 11 hours during the night. Depending on when you start sleep training, your baby might not wake you up much during the night. If you have not started sleep training or continuing the process, your baby might still wake you up once or twice. Many babies are capable of sleeping through the night at this point with an occasional middle of the night awakening to be fed. They will begin to transition from needing their afternoon nap at eight months old.

8 to 15 Months

Between 8 to 15 months of age, your baby should sleep between 13 to 14 ½ hours in a 24-hour period. Without their afternoon nap, they will still have a morning and midday nap. Their morning nap will last about one and a half hours and their midday nap two to two and a half hours. They will sleep a total of nine to 11 ½ hours during the night. Once your baby is about 14 months old, their morning nap will disappear.

16 to 36 Months

Between 16 to 36 months of age, your baby should sleep a total of 11 ½ to 13 hours in a 24-hour period. Down to only one nap—their midday nap—they will sleep between one and a half to two and a half hours. You do not want them sleeping more during the day unless they are sick, because it will be harder for them to sleep at night. During the night, they should sleep nine to 11 ½ hours. Once they are 36 months old, they will no longer have a midday nap, unless they are really tired.

What Does Healthy Sleep Look Like?

You will notice a significant change in your baby's temperament just after one healthy night/day of sleep. They will wake cheerful and alert. They will smile and coo. They will be more curious and bright-eyed and in a quiet alert state.

This quiet alert state refers to the time your baby awakes but is not fussing or in need of anything. This time typically occurs just after your baby wakes up. You will notice they seem to be in deep thought or contemplating the world around them. They are simply taking in everything they see. The time your baby spends in this quiet alert state can have an impact on their ability to learn and develop properly. When your baby has had a long or even short periods of quality sleep, this quiet and alert state becomes a regular fixture in their sleeping routine.

Infants who do not nap or sleep for long periods of time tend to skip this quiet alert state frequently. They will wake up still feeling groggy, tired, and irritable. This is why many babies will wake up and immediately begin to scream or cry.

Understanding Sleep Problems

Regular sleep disturbances have several negative effects on your baby's mood and learning abilities. There a number of factors that can cause sleep problems, which range from mild disturbances to severe sleep disorders, all of which can often be corrected with the implementation of a healthy sleep schedule. Knowing and understanding how sleep disturbances can affect your baby will allow you to identify any serious red flags. If you ever feel your baby is suffering from a sleep disorder, contact their pediatrician immediately. While you may understand what these disorders are, your baby's doctor can help formulate a more appropriate treatment plan and provide you with the necessary resources that can better help your baby get more sleep.

Common Sleep Disorders

- **Dyssomnias.** These types of sleep disorders revolve around having difficulty falling asleep and staying asleep. The most common types of dyssomnias disorder include sleep apnea, restless leg syndrome, periodic limb movement, and insomnia.

- **Parasomnias.** Parasomnias disorders involve abnormal activities that occur while sleeping. The two most common types of disorders associated with parasomnias include sleepwalking and night terrors.

There are also psychiatric disorders that can be caused by sleep issues and additional medical disorders that can be impairing your child's ability to sleep. Again, if you have any concerns, no matter how small, about your child's sleep, do not hesitate to consult with their doctor to address your concerns.

Also, keep in mind that other factors can contribute to your child being unable to sleep. Teething, growth spurts, and illness can regularly cause sleep disturbance.

Understand Your Child's Sleeping Cues and Patterns

When your baby reaches about three months, they will begin to give more cues and signs that they are getting sleepy. The most common cues include:

- Yawning
- Not wanting to play
- Rubbing eyes
- Clenched fists
- Waving their arms or legs about or having jerky movements
- Becoming fussy
- Making sleeping sounds
- Beginning to cry
- Pulling on their face or grimacing
- Looking away from people or objects

These cues let you know that they should be laid down for a nap. Missing these cues can cause your baby to become overactive, which results in more difficulty getting them to nap or sleep at night. Additionally, your baby may have a glazed look in their eyes that shows they are overtired or they may cry more frequently.

Key Points to Remember

- The amount of sleep your baby needs will decrease as they grow. Up until your child is around 18 months old, they will maintain a nap schedule that consists of at least two naps.
- Many internal and external factors can hinder your child's sleep. Never hesitate to contact your child's doctor to address these concerns.
- From the age of three months old, your baby will begin to give you sleep cues. Pay attention to these cues so you know when your baby needs to sleep.

CHAPTER 2: The Importance of Healthy Sleeping

Healthy sleeping patterns do not just make for a happier baby; in fact, it is crucial that your baby gets into a healthy sleeping routine early on. When your child is not getting enough sleep, it can have an impact on their ability to learn, their cognitive development, and a number of other factors depending on their age. Let's take a look at some of the key factors that can be delayed when a child does not learn healthy sleeping habits.

Effects of Healthy Sleep

Sleep will affect your child differently as they grow. When your baby does not get adequate sleep, this could set them back from reaching major milestones in their development.

0 to 3 Months

Infants at this early age need to be getting adequate sleep so they are able to learn more when they are awake. Children who take longer naps when they are infants will often find it easier to learn as they get older. During the first three months, your baby will sleep a majority of the time. It is in this sleep that your baby is actually learning the most.

Babies at this age who do not get proper sleep will be fussier when they are awake. This can lead to mom or dad having to comfort their child throughout the day. It can be more challenging to get your baby to settle down when it is time to sleep at night. The combination of baby not sleeping and the constant need for rocking and soothing activities during the day can cause major strain on the parents and interrupt their ability to get sleep and feel well-rested. This, as a result, puts a strain on the relationship between baby and parent. It can be more difficult for mothers to bond with their infants when they are not getting the right amount of sleep.

3 to 5 Months

Babies at this age should be settling into a regular sleeping pattern. This can alleviate some stress for mom and dad and can make fitting in daily activities more easily. From birth to about five to six months of age, your baby will be doing most of their learning and development while they are asleep. During sleep, your baby's nervous system is forming connections between the brain and various muscles in their body. You may notice this occurring when you baby twitches in their sleep. Proper sleep is also vital for proper growth and weight gain during this time. As I mentioned before, my son was in the lower weight percentile, even though he was feeding all the time. When he actually began to sleep his body was able to properly use energy to help him grow and gain weight.

From as early as three months of age, babies will begin making word correlations to objects around them, such as being able to identify their mom's or dad's face when they see them. A baby who is not getting enough sleep will have more difficulty developing these word pairings and connections and will struggle even more with being able to remember or recall these associations.

During the three to five-month range, difficulty sleeping can begin to affect your baby's development significantly. This is when you may notice your child in a calm and alert state just after waking when they have had a good night's sleep. It is also during this time that your baby should be sleeping for longer periods of time overnight. Many parents have success with getting their baby to sleep through the night or at least through a majority of the night with only one or two feedings.

Babies who are not acquiring the proper amount of sleep at this age will be less approachable. They will not want to interact with others or the things in their surroundings. When they withdraw from daily activities like this, they are missing out on vital learning opportunities and gaining socialization skills.

Unfortunately, there are several factors that can hinder your baby's sleep patterns at this age. Just when your baby begins to settle into a routine, they may begin teething or go through a period of sleep regression. It is still important to provide your baby with the comfort and security they need to help them best get the right amount of sleep each night.

Signs your baby is not getting enough sleep at this age can include:

- Only being able to sleep for a short amount of time, usually between 40 to 60 minutes.
- Struggling to fall asleep quickly.
- Becoming fussier as the day progresses.
- Startling easily by the things around them.
- Being quick to cry and becoming upset easily.

5 to 8 Months

At this age, children are really beginning to adapt their sleep patterns. They are learning how to soothe themselves to sleep. It is also around this time that nap times will begin to change a great deal with fewer naps during the day. How a child sleeps during these months will often reflect in their behavior and learning abilities as they get older. Babies who get adequate sleep at this age are able to remember what they learn, even if they are unable to communicate it at this time to their parents. When your baby is sleeping enough, they will be alert and interested in daily activities with you and other family members. A baby who is sleep-deprived, even by just a small amount of sleep, will be inattentive and uninterested in what is going on around them. Babies who do not get enough sleep will have more difficulty making generalizations and developing the skills for word recognition, and this will affect their ability to recall new information they may have just learned.

Getting proper sleep allows your baby to stay alert in activities during the day. They will be able to focus more on learning new word pairings and correlation through different activities. However, if your child is not getting proper sleep, they may be too irritable to enjoy these learning experiences and may be unable to fully develop the skills to make word-object associations.

Children who wake too much during their longer sleep periods at night can often develop less sensory tolerance. This low sensory threshold can result in constant sensory seeking or avoidance behavior that will make even the simplest task in the day seem like a battle. Sensory issues can include sensitivity to lights, sounds, noise, smell, and touch. These issues can result in difficulty feeding, learning to speak, mood regulation, and a range of behavioral and developmental obstacles.

Separation anxiety may become a factor in sleep challenges at this age. When added to the cognitive and motor development your baby is reaching, these all can add up to serious sleep disturbances for your baby.

The signs for poor sleep at this age:

- Falling asleep immediately after being placed in their car seat.
- Irritability.
- Not engaging in play activities.
- Being increasingly fussy.
- Seeming more bothered by sounds, lights, or sudden movements.

8 to 15 Months

Your baby should be sleeping through the night by this time. Keep in mind that it is common for babies to wake up frequently throughout the night and drift back to sleep up to six times. If your baby is waking in the middle of the night and not soothing themselves back to sleep at this point, this negatively impacts the amount and quality of sleep they are getting. When a child screams for their parents in the middle of the night regularly between eight to 15 months, they are developing poor sleeping habits. This will negatively impact their ability to adopt a healthy sleep pattern later on, which will begin to affect their behavior and temperament significantly.

During these months, your baby is developing their mobile skills, such as sitting up on their own, crawling, or walking even! This is an exciting time for your baby as they are able to move around and see their surroundings from a different perspective. They are having many new experiences every day, and as exciting as this is, this can impact your child's ability and desire to sleep.

This is also the time when babies will begin to incorporate more solid foods into their diets and bottle or breastfeeding may begin to reduce. Changes in diet and feedings along with their determination to master their new skills can trigger a variety of sleep disturbances.

16 to 36 Months

Children at this age may not be napping for as long or as often as they once did. Naps are still an important time for children at this age. When children nap well, they are able to adjust to different circumstances with ease. This can make transitioning from activities less stressful, and for many, this will make the transition to a more structured school setting an easier phase.

Children who tend to nap for short spurts or not at all at this age will all suffer from more night wakings. Many children at this age who have poor sleeping habits have developed these habits from a very early age. Most children will form clear sleep routines at this age, which have been acquired since they were about five months old. If your baby is used to you rocking and soothing them to sleep, they will expect and need this to get them to doze off. If you baby is used to waking every few hours for feeding, they will continue to awake after just a few hours even if they do not need to be fed. The effect of poor sleep may not give you clear signs at first, but when they reach this age, you will notice their temperament is less pleasant and they become more difficult.

Do Not Forget About Yourself

As a mother, I completely understand how easy it is to forget about yourself. You are embarrassed to tell people how many days it has been since you have showered. You do not want to admit that you are irritable because you are tired. After all, everyone knows that this is part of motherhood, especially with a little one. It is something that you just have to accept, right? Wrong! You should never believe when society treats the lack of sleep mothers get as "part of the job." Here is the real factor—if you do not get the sleep you need to take care of yourself, you cannot properly take care of your baby. You cannot focus and this can cause you to make mistakes or potentially (I do not like bringing this up, but it has happened thousands of times to moms all over the world) harm your baby. There are stories of babies slipping from their mother's arms, mothers not fully paying attention when they are changing their baby's diaper and the baby rolls off the changing table or couch. There are even stories of mothers falling asleep while driving their vehicles because they are exhausted.

It is not easy, especially at first, but you and your baby need to get quality sleep from the moment they are born. If this means you need to ask people for help; please, ask people for help. There are many people in your life that would love to help you, from family members to friends to fellow-moms in community groups. I know you think that you need to do everything for your baby and you do not want to think of someone else taking care of your precious little one, even for a few hours. But it is more important that you take care of yourself so you can do the best for your baby.

Effects of Sleep Deprivation

You feel like you haven't slept in days—it is like being awake forever. Your mental, emotional, and physical health is not as strong as it used to be because you are so exhausted. In fact, if there was a medal of dedication for a mother who has not slept since her baby (or first baby) was born, you would be the recipient. While this means you are doing what you need to do to meet the needs of your little one, this can have some serious negative consequences for both you and your baby. Mothers who lack the proper amount of sleep are not able to fully attend to their children, though most have perfected the ability to function optimally on very little sleep.

Your baby can also suffer severely from sleep deprivation. It is essential that you take note of the warning signs you or your baby may be exhibiting that indicate you are being deprived of sleep. It is also equally important that you take to heart these red flags and make adjustments to ensure you and/or your baby is sleeping soundly.

When You Are Sleep Deprived

Regularly neglecting to get the proper amount of sleep nightly can put you at greater risk for a number of health issues and not just having a poor mood. Those who regularly get fewer than five hours of sleep a night have a higher risk of developing type 2 diabetes, struggle with obesity, suffer from cardiovascular disease, and feel more depressed. These are all factors that will not only hinder your quality of life, but they will also hinder your ability to properly care for your child in the way you want. As a mother, you are already at a slightly greater risk for many of these health issues; skimming out on sleep increases this risk even more.

When you are not getting the proper amount of sleep, your brain singles the body to obtain more energy from food. Since your body is not reenergizing when you sleep, it needs to find a different way to be able to properly function. This can lead to an increase in weight, which leads to many of the health issues just mentioned. For moms, this is especially problematic. Since many women already struggle with their weight and confidence after giving birth, this excess food intake will only make the struggle more challenging. Postpartum depression is not uncommon for women to develop after giving birth because they are unable to or cannot balance taking care of their new baby as they want with taking care of themselves. One of the first things a parent will sacrifice to take care of their child and balance all their other responsibilities is sleep.

Chronic sleep deprivation affects every aspect of your life. You may notice that you are more forgetful and you are more indecisive. Lack of sleep makes it especially difficult to focus on what is happening around you. You are more likely to forget where you put things, what someone has just said to you, appointments, and much more. Problem-solving is also a task as your brain's processing speeds have slowed down a great deal. These problems can affect your time-management, which increases your stress levels that, in turn, fuels your exhaustion.

You will notice that it is not just your memory and problem-solving skills that are hindered but your motor skills and emotional regulation gets thrown off as well. You may find that you lose your balance or feel dizzy more often. You notice that your emotions take control of the situation and can cause minor hiccups in your day, completely derailing you and sending you into an emotional fit. When you are lacking sleep, your body and brain are unable to react appropriately. This is what causes your motor skills to get out of sync since the signals from your brain to the rest of your body are not getting sent out in time so that you avoid bumping into furniture or tripping over your own feet. The overreaction of emotion caused by sleep deprivation can cause serious strain on many of your relationships, including the one you share with your baby.

When Your Baby Is Sleep Deprived

If sleep-deprivation has so many negative effects on you as an adult, just imagine the turmoil it can cause your young baby. When your baby is sleep deprived, you will notice a change in their mood and temperament first. They will be fussier, cry more, and be uninterested in their surroundings. Often, they will be quickly irritated by noises or lights in their surroundings. But there are additional signs that can indicate your baby is not getting the proper sleep on a regular basis.

Babies who sleep less than the suggested amount will show little interest in the things around them. In fact, babies who are sleep deprived will often try to avoid stimulating objects or activities.

Sleep deprivation can be a serious safety concern for children who are just learning to move about on their own. Just as being sleep deprived can cause you to become more accident prone, so it can cause your baby to be so as well. When you add in their poor coordination and balance skills at a young age with the poor motor skills they will additionally have due to improper sleep, your child can become seriously injured.

Many children who lack proper sleep will also become very clingy or needy with their parents. You may notice your child holds onto your legs when they are up and about or they constantly scream to have you pick them up and carry them wherever you go. This can be a clear sign of sleep deprivation.

Oddly, sleep deprivation can also increase your baby's hyperactivity when it is closer to bedtime. This then creates the cycle of your little one having more difficulty falling asleep, staying asleep, and then not getting enough sleep; this cycle continually repeats.

Sleep deprivation can lead to children being unable to recover from their emotions or be able to regulate their emotions. This should not be a surprise as you probably have already experienced yourself how lack of sleep can make it more difficult for you to remain calm and patient throughout the day. Serious and frequent sleep issues will also make it difficult to feed your child. Children that are often labeled as picky eaters will more often than not be suffering from poor sleep routines than they are from not wanting to eat what is in front of them.

Key Points to Remember

- Sleep affects your baby's development, can impair their ability to learn, and can result in them missing crucial milestones.
- Sleep deprivation can be harmful to mom as well as baby.
- When mom is sleep-deprived, she is more likely to misplace things, become forgetful, and be unable to fully concentrate or focus while caring for a baby.
- Sleep deprivation affects your baby in similar ways as it affects you. Your baby will be more fussy, irritable, and unable to retain new information that is vital for their growth.

CHAPTER 3: Your Baby's First Months – What to Expect and How to Start Implementing Healthy Sleep Practices

As soon as your baby is born, they will go through a number of changes. Mom and dad are going through changes as well, as they adapt to having a little one in the house. In the time from when your baby is born to about one month, your baby is still used to the comfort and safety of mom's womb. They are, and will continue to be, completely dependent on their caregivers to provide them with their every need. This time-frame, known as the fourth trimester, can be exhausting for first-time moms not used to feeding, changing, burping, and rocking their newborn for what seems like all day long. After this time period, your baby begins to make clear classifications such as recognizing when it is night or day and beginning to regulate their sleep cycle. Understanding what your baby needs from you during this fourth trimester and up until they are three months old will help you introduce healthy sleep patterns for your baby such as sleeping in their crib. During this time, it is vital that mom learns how to get the sleep she is missing out because of the constant night feedings and awakenings.

What Is the Fourth Trimester?

The fourth trimester refers to the time from when your baby is born through their first three months. During this time, some changes will occur with your baby and they will begin to make adjustments as they interact and see the world around them. Your baby will be developing their senses, controlling reflexes, and also learning to respond to their environment and the people in it.

During the first three months of your baby's arrival, a great deal of development will occur both mentally and physically. Your baby will need to adjust to all the new noises, smells, sights, and more that they never experienced inside the womb. Temperature changes, the feeling of their clothing, and other stimulates will begin to affect your baby in ways they will need to learn to adjust to.

During the fourth trimester, your baby relies a great deal on others to care for them. Additionally, it is the parents who need to supply enough attention, love, and care to their new baby to help them develop proper attraction and security skills.

During the fourth trimester, your baby will develop a number of necessary skills, such as:

- Controlling their breathing
- Adopting sleep and feeding patterns
- Being able to sleep with distraction or outside noise
- Learning to self-sooth
- Learning to cry out for attention to get needs met
- Beginning to interact with family members or objects
- Learning to distinguish between night and day

When you provide your baby with what they need at this time, they will be able to quickly acquire these new skills.

What Are Your Baby's Needs During the Fourth Trimester?

Throughout the fourth trimester, your baby will need a great deal of support as they adjust to all the newness of their world. Where before they could relax in the comfort of your womb, they now have wide spaces around them. All the new information they obtain will be absorbed like a sponge, which will benefit them as they grow even more over the next few months. Your baby will need a lot of stimulation during this time to ensure the proper connections in the brain are being made. There are a number of ways you can help promote your baby's development and assist them with adjusting to their new worlds:

1. **Provide your baby with skin-to-skin interaction**. When you notice your baby is especially fussy during these first few months, this could be a result of needing to feel the same comfort they felt when you were carrying them. Skin-to-skin interaction will give your baby the comfort of a familiar smell and the sound of your heartbeat. These smells and your heartbeat can help them regulate their own heartbeat. Skin-to-skin holding will also encourage latching if you are breastfeeding.
2. **Feed your baby when they are hungry.** For the first three months, your baby will eat frequently. This is because their stomachs are still much too small to hold a significant amount of food. When your baby cries, you want to provide them with the nourishment they need. Feeding on demand will give you the reassurance that your baby's dietary needs are being met and that you are providing them with the right amount of fuel they require.
3. **Swaddle your baby.** Your baby, from the time they are born up until about three months, may need to be swaddled in order for them to rest properly. For the past nine months or so they have been used to sleeping in a confined and tight space. They will still need to feel this pressure when they fall asleep. Swaddling your baby will help them transition into a better

sleeping schedule and will provide them with the comfort necessary for them to sleep soundly. Keep in mind that if your baby is at the age where they are able to flip from their back to stomach, you should no longer be swaddling your baby to sleep for safety concerns. Always remember to check on your baby when you swaddle them to ensure they have not accidentally rolled onto their bellies.

4. **Wear your baby**. Your baby has been used to being swung around, bounced, and having constant movement. It is likely that laying still for long periods of time can be distressing for your baby. Many babies will become fussy for what appears to be no reason multiple times a day. If your baby is not hungry or tired, it is very likely that they miss this constant movement. Wearing your baby will soothe your fussy baby and can help them drift to sleep.

Introducing Routines Into Your Baby's Life

There is a debate on how soon you can start introducing routines into your baby's life. Some experts state you can start a couple of weeks after you bring them home from the hospital while others believe the best time to start is at three months of age. By this time your baby understands there is a difference between day and night, giving you an upper hand when it comes to establishing their routines. Another advantage of waiting until they are three months old is because they have learned a few self-soothing strategies to help them learn to independently fall asleep.

Developing routines can help both you and your baby in many ways. Adequate sleep is a key reason that many moms and dads want to establish routines early on. This isn't just to ensure their baby is getting enough sleep but because the parents need sleep too. When you begin setting up regular routines, you can start small with a few necessary structure times and then add more as your baby makes the proper adjustments.

Daytime Routine

You can begin to teach your baby that daytime is different from night time by establishing routines early on. Some of the ways you can begin teaching your child these differences include:

- Opening the curtains or blinds in their room as soon as they wake up.
- Not trying to limit or avoid making noise when your baby naps during the day.
- Filling your baby's day with a lot of playtime and activities.
- Beginning to take note of when they need a nap and how long these naps last.

Nighttime Routine

Establishing a nighttime sleep routine at this young age will help your baby better recognize and understand the difference between night and day. This will also help them make the connection that nighttime is for sleeping. When beginning to establish a nighttime routine, it is helpful to follow these simple guidelines:

1. Dim or lower the lights.
2. Keep your voice low when talking to your baby and try not to talk too much.
3. Avoid any play activities with your baby just before it is time for them to sleep.
4. Once you have fed and changed your baby, lay them down in

their crib.
5. Try to avoid middle-of-the-night diaper changes. If you do need to change your baby in the middle of the night, do not turn on the lights; instead, use a dim flashlight or night light and change your baby as quickly as possible.

Your Baby's Crib Is More Important Than You Think

During the fourth trimester, your baby will seemingly be able to sleep through just about anything and sleep anywhere. Most often your baby will fall asleep in your arms as you rock them to sleep or as they are feeding.

If your baby frequently falls asleep as you are holding them, this is a habit that can be challenging to break as they grow. Instead, lay your baby down in their crib when they are still awake but drowsy. This will help your baby begin to learn how to fall asleep without the need of you rocking or holding them sleep.

"Sleeping When Your Baby Sleeps" Is Just an Idea

You will hear and have probably heard the number one advice given to moms is to sleep when their baby sleeps. If your baby is napping, you should take this time to nap as well. This advice is given for good reason. Most moms will lose a significant amount of sleep after their baby is born, so it is vital that they are able to make up for sleep lost during the evening hours at some point in the day. With frequent feeds and even throughout the night, diaper changes, or merely screaming fits, you will be with your little one a great deal.

Most mothers, however, skip the naps to catch up on housework and other responsibilities. They tend to keep running themselves until empty, and even then, they will run on whatever fumes they can muster to find. If you are breastfeeding, it is even more challenging to abide by this "sleep when your baby sleeps" rule. When your baby is sleeping, you will often be pumping breast milk. While this idea is nice in reality, it is just not possible for many moms to abide by.

In order for you to get the sleep you desperately need as well, you will need to establish a routine for yourself that will allow you to get in some rest when your baby naps once in a while. If possible, create a schedule with your partner where they are able to take over some of the feedings or early morning changes so you can catch up on sleep. Also, never be afraid to reach out to friends and family members who can watch your little one for a few hours so you can rest and recharge.

Key Points to Remember

- The fourth trimester is a time of significant development and growth for your baby.
- Your baby will need you to provide them with the same comforts they had in the womb such as being swaddled or hearing your heartbeat.
- Begin to introduce healthy sleep habits by establishing simple daytime and evening routines. This will help teach your baby the difference between night and day and will also allow them to recognize that the night is a time for sleeping.
- The safest place for your baby to sleep is in their own crib.

CHAPTER 4: The Importance of Answering Your Baby's Cry – Is There a No-Cry Method?

There are dozens of methods you can try when it comes to sleep training your baby. However, most of the methods fall into two types of categories. The first is known as the no-cry or the no-tears method. The second is known as the cry-it-out method. Both methods have their benefits, disadvantages, experts, and debates among parents. The key to remember is that you always want to go with your instincts. Your baby will tell you when one sleep method is not working and when you should try another.

Is There a No-Cry Method to Sleep Training?

The no-cry method, which is sometimes referred to as the no-tears method, is believed to be a false method by many people because there is crying when it comes to sleep training. In a way, this is true. Your baby will cry because this is the main way they communicate with you to let you know that they need something. The no-cry method to sleep training does not mean there will be no tears; it means there will be a gradual transition to your baby's sleep routine that will result in fewer tears, and most importantly, you will not leave your baby alone to cry.

The no-cry method establishes a nighttime routine so your baby can learn to expect what is coming next just before they settle down for their overnight slumber. This method helps you and baby develop quiet and comforting rituals so that your baby's needs are met and there will be less crying and fussing when you lay them down.

Benefits of the No-Tears Method

Create a nurturing bedtime routine. The no-tears method helps create a positive association with sleep. This nurturing routine will allow your baby to know they are safe and secure, so there is no need to panic when mom or dad is not there if they happen to wake in the middle of the night. This allows you to gently teach your baby to self-soothe while they sleep on their own.

Establishing a No-Tears Method Routine

Creating a routine with the no-tears method will take time. Learning what works best for you and your baby is not going to be an overnight accomplishment. Just as with everything else your baby will learn, it takes consistency and time to guide your baby into a soothing and positive sleeping pattern. While it takes more time, the trade-off can result in a happier, well-rested baby that is able to soothe themselves to sleep in the long term. The no-cry method is not a one-size-fits-all; each parent approaches this sleeping method in a way that feels best for them. The following tips can guide you through establishing a bedtime routine where there are fewer tears and more sleep for you and your baby:

1. **Be consistent with daytime naps.** When your baby is on a regular daytime napping schedule, it will allow for the nighttime sleep to go much smoother.
2. **Don't try to keep your baby up late in hopes they will sleep longer through the night.** It is typical for babies to fall asleep at a much earlier time, around 7:00 p.m. when they are only a few months old. When you are beginning to establish a bedtime

sleep routine, you want to start by putting your baby to bed earlier in the evening. Keeping your baby up later will only result in an overtired baby, and this will make falling asleep for them much more difficult. With the no-tears method, you want to avoid trying to get your baby to sleep when they are upset. Putting them to bed earlier can help you avoid an overtired and unhappy baby.

3. **Be consistent with your bedtime routine.** You want to do the same activities every night. These activities should be soothing and help your baby relax and prepare for sleep. Feed your baby, bathe them, read to them, and then put them to sleep. Do the same thing every night so that your baby gets used to the schedule of events that leads up to their long night's sleep.

4. **Establish verbal cues that will remind your baby it is bedtime.** You can come up with a phrase such as "It's time to go night, night" or "It's sleepy time" to say out loud to your baby so they can begin to associate these words with bedtime. You can also have a specific sound or song you hum that will put your baby in sleep mode.

5. **Tailor your baby's sleep environment to their own comfort.** You may notice your baby sleeps longer when they have quiet sounds playing in the background or your baby may need their sleep environment to be a bit darker. Whatever your baby prefers to help them sleep longer, you want to set their environment to reflect what they need. Having a comfortable and relaxing sleep environment will result in a longer, more quality sleep for your baby.

6. **Learn when your baby is crying because they need something from you.** Babies will make plenty of noise as they sleep; they may even cry out a few times, then quickly fall back into their slumber. You want to be able to understand what sounds your

baby makes and not be so quick to rush in to soothe your baby back to sleep. The goal is to help them learn to fall back to sleep on their own and this can only be accomplished if they are left undisturbed to do so. If your baby whimpers or cries in the middle of the night, allow them some time to self-soothe before you check on them.

The Cry-It-Out Method

The cry-it-out method (CIO) is one sleep training method that carries a great deal of controversy. This method is implemented to varying degrees, the most extreme being your child is left to cry themselves to sleep for however long that takes. On the less extreme side, you allow your baby to cry in their room for 5 minutes at bedtime before you rush in to give them a sweet pat on the head, maybe a kiss, and then say good-night, and walk out of the room. When your baby starts to scream and cry again, you let them go for a little longer and so on until they fall asleep.

With any sleep training method there is bound to be tears. It should be expected that your baby will have some difficulty transitioning from being rocked and lulled to sleep in the arms of their parents to being placed in a crib or bassinet. This is also why most babies wake up in the middle of the night crying out. They fall asleep in the safe comfort of the arms of their parents and they suddenly wake up with no one around. This can be a frightening experience.

Though many sleep training methods involve crying, these methods are not the same as the cry-it-out method. With other sleep training methods, you put your baby to bed when they are beginning to show you signs of being tired. There can be crying as your baby is not used to being laid in their bed to sleep, but you do not leave them in their crib to cry. You stand by them and comfort them and help soothe them to sleep. This reassures them that they are safe. You leave the room after they have fallen asleep in their crib. If they wake up and begin to cry after you have left the room, there is a short wait period before parents re-enter their room. This wait period is rarely over 5 minutes.

The cry-it-out method, on the other hand, may suggest putting you baby to bed when they are happily playing. You allow them to play in their bed for a little and you leave the room as they do so. This is often the immediate cause for the screaming to begin. The parents are then to wait at least 5 minutes before returning in the room to say goodnight and leave quickly. They then sit outside the room for 10 minutes before entering. This continues until the child falls asleep. This is not a highly recommended method for sleep training; though it may work for a few parents, there are some long-term effects that can cause the parent-child relationship to be hindered.

What to Know About the Cry-It-Out Method

1. This is not an easy approach to sleep training. Having to listen to your baby cry for extended periods of time is more challenging for the parent than it is for the baby most times.
2. During the first few days, your baby can cry from anywhere between 15 minutes and up to an hour in many cases. This can be very nerve-racking for parents and is the reason why many do not follow through with the process after the first try.
3. If you revert back to previous ways of soothing your baby to sleep, for instance by feeding and rocking to sleep, you will most likely need to start the whole process over again.
4. Some say that this method can help babies learn to handle stress better. Since they are able to work through the stressful situation of not having someone there to rock them to sleep,

this can carry over to them being able to manage stress as they grow older in more efficient ways.

5. This method won't eliminate crying every single night. Many babies will need to cry for a few minutes each time they are put to sleep, including naps.
6. This method is not for everyone. Allowing your baby to cry it out might not result in more quality sleep for your baby.
7. While this method may begin teaching your baby how to manage stress, this doesn't necessarily mean their brains will not be affected by the stress in the moment. When your baby is crying, their cortisol levels will rise. Cortisol is a stress hormone that the body naturally produces and releases. If your baby is crying for long periods of time, this can cause an excess amount of cortisol being released, which can cause an imbalance in their system. When your baby wakes, these cortisol levels can still be high and this can affect your baby in the day time hours. This increase cortisol can make it difficult for them to nap during the day. You will notice more behavioral issues such as becoming easily frustrated, throwing things, or biting. You may also find it more difficult to soothe you baby when they are upset.
8. This method does not allow for a strong bonding experience. Your baby may not feel as safe or secure with you when you allow them to cry it out. When your baby is crying, they are screaming for you because they need something. Even though it is just to rock or soothe them to sleep, your baby may associate you not rushing in to lull them to sleep with not being able to trust you when they are in need of something else. There is a chance that your baby may not look at you as a trusted protector.
9. Prolonged intense screaming may result in your baby having

more difficulty when they are older and how they handle trauma. The screaming that can occur with the cry-it-out method may damage some neural connections in the brain, which can leave them hypersensitive to any trauma they encounter later in life.

10. If you are breastfeeding, this method might throw off your milk production. If you are not rushing in to feed your baby in the middle of the night, you are going longer periods of time without feeding. Breast milk is produced when feeding occurs, so when you cut back on the feeding, there will be a decrease in the milk you will produce.
11. The intense crying can last for long periods of time and occur multiple times a night, which can cause your baby's blood pressure to rise. Just as high-blood pressure in adults can lead to long-term complications, it is no different in babies. Prolonged high-blood pressure can cause damage to the kidney's and can affect how the blood vessels in the body develops. This results in the heart having to continuously do double the work to pump blood to the major organs.
12. This method should never be used with babies who are 3 months or younger.

The major concern that parents and professionals have with this method of sleep training is simply leaving your baby to cry alone. While crying is inevitable, parents find it especially challenging to sit by their baby's door and allow them to scream and cry alone in their room without providing them with any form of comfort or reassurance that they are safe. This method is not recommended as an effective form of sleep training. The sleep training process should allow parent and child to maintain their nurturing bond and feelings of security. This method can often negatively affect this parental bond.

Answering Your Baby's Cries

For any of the sleep training methods to be a success, you first need to understand how your baby cries. You may have noticed that the way your baby cries when they are hungry sounds a great deal different from how they cry when they need a diaper change or when they are tired. Every baby will have a fluctuation in their crying cues. When you become more aware and observe the way your baby cries, you will be able to implement any of the sleep training methods with more ease and confidence, as you will be able to tell if your baby needs something more than just being rocked to sleep.

Types of Cries

1. When your baby is hungry, they will cry a certain way but will also indicate with specific movements of the body that they need to be fed. Your baby may have a more low-pitched cry that is repetitive and rhythmic. Your baby will also perform a sucking motion with their tongue or purse their lips together. If you are breastfeeding, you will notice your baby reaching up in search of your breast. When your baby is crying when they are hungry, you want to respond quickly and supply them with food. If you wait too long to feed your baby after they have started crying to be fed, they can have more difficulty feeding when you do try.
2. Your baby will have a nasal-focused and continuous cry when they are feeling uncomfortable or getting tired. This cry will intensify and your baby may rub their eyes, yawn, or tug at their ear. Your baby may also need to have a diaper change when you hear this type of cry.
3. Your baby will have a fussy or whiny cry when they have had enough of something, either with feeding or when doing

certain play activities like tummy time. Along with the fussy whine, your baby will often turn away from what they don't want any more or make hand-arm movements that indicate they have had enough.

4. When your baby is bored, you will hear your baby cry out in coos. This is to get positive attention when they are not getting the interaction they are looking for; these cooing cries will turn into more whiny cries or fussiness. If your baby is still not actively engaged when the fussiness occurs, they will begin to cry out in louder, shorter spurts that will often be followed by whimpers.

5. A baby who is suffering from colic will exhibit intense and extreme cries. They will also fidget and squirm a great deal as they scream and in between screams. The main difference between a colic cry and most other cries is they can last for hours without relief. No matter what you try, your baby may not settle for a while. When you are noticing these types of screams with your baby, you want to try to provide as much comfort as possible with the understanding that the wailing will most likely continue despite all your efforts. Try to lay your baby on their tummy or across your lap and gently rub their backs.

6. You will notice that your baby's cry will sound different when they are sick as well. When your baby is sick, you will hear a more nasal or congested cry. These cries will often begin as low whimpers and the cry will be more low-pitched than the other cries you have experienced. When your baby is sick, you want to comfort them as best as you can. This may not be an ideal time to try any sleep training methods as you want to ensure your baby is sleeping quickly and easily without additional discomforts.

Additionally, your baby will cry differently when they are too hot or cold or when they may be getting overstimulated from some sensory input in their environments such as the lights or sound. Your baby will also cry differently when they simply need a change in scenery. Before you begin to sleep train your baby, it is best that you are able to distinguish between the various cries.

Keep in mind that there are some cries that you will not be able to identify what your baby needs. With newborn babies, it is very likely that you will have a number of crying episodes where you cannot pinpoint a trigger for. This type of crying session can be from a long fun-filled day or from excess stress you are unaware of. Just as you will have days where you are simply exhausted and your energy levels are tapped out, your baby will have these days as well.

Tips for Understanding Your Baby's Cries

Establishing a routine will help you better determine what your baby's cries mean. When your baby gets into a regular daytime routine and they begin to cry when it is usually feeding time, you will discover and be able to identify this type of cry when they are hungry.

Remember to stay calm and patient. When you encounter a crying spell that you are unable to find a solution for, this can cause you to stress out and become frantic. Take a breath and understand it is completely normal for many babies to cry for unknown reasons. If you are concerned about your baby's crying episode, it is better to speak to a pediatrician. They can better help you understand what may be causing the crying episodes and this can help alleviate any additional stress you may be feeling because your initial thought will automatically conclude that something is seriously wrong with them.

During crying episodes where you have tried everything possible to calm your baby, you want to allow yourself a break. It is okay to step out on the front porch for a few deep breaths of air. Ensure that your baby is safe in their crib or bassinet and allow yourself a moment to regain your composure and calm your nerves. While you want to be a supermom, you also need to admit that you do have limits. Even the best of moms will find themselves becoming frustrated when they are unable to soothe their crying baby. Do not try to force yourself to fight through the frustration. It is much safer for you and your baby if you take a break for a few minutes so you can come back to them with a clearer and calmer mindset.

Key Point to Remember

- Babies cry. There is no method that will completely eliminate crying for the bedtime routine.
- The no-cry method helps establish healthy sleep routines that your baby can carry with them for the rest of their lives.
- The cry-it-out method is an extreme form of sleep training that may teach your baby to self-soothe but can also have long-term negative effects, and as such, is not recommended.
- Whichever method you choose, it is your choice to make.
- Crying is the only way your baby knows how to communicate with you. By understanding their different types of cries, you will better understand what your baby needs and is asking for.

CHAPTER 5: There Is No One Baby, There Is No One Book

Even when sleep training is going well, you can still run into challenges and feel frustrated. For me, this happened with my first-born. He would go to sleep when his father or grandmother put him down, but he would not react in the same manner when I put him to bed. I would place him in his crib, just like my husband and mother would, but he would still cry. He would cry a lot and I could not stand hearing him cry like he did. I could not understand why it took him so long to fall asleep when I put him to bed.

I contacted a friend of mine who had gone through the sleep training process. With frustration in my voice, I told her, "I do not understand what I am doing wrong! I am doing everything by the book. It works fine with my husband, but not with me!"

My friend calmly responded, "Grace, there is no book to tell you how to do anything with your baby. They each have their own book and your baby's book is different than my baby's book. They are individuals and have different needs. They will respond to everything in a different way. You have to create your own "book" to make this work by responding to his needs."

This became the moment where everything changed for me. I did not look at sleep training as a "what not to do" list. Instead, I looked at it as a "follow what my baby needs" guidelines list. The fact is I gave my baby a little more TLC than my husband and this is what he needed from me when I put him to bed. Once I started following my baby's cues and what he needed, the rejection started to wind down. Soon, bedtime was quality time for us and the process went a lot smoother.

Every Baby Is Different

Sometimes parents forget that our precious little ones are individuals. We get deep into the thought of "what the book said" or "what worked for my friend" and forget that our baby is unique, and that we need to follow what our baby is telling us the best we can to help him or her thrive. It is a process that often takes trial, error, some tears but also a plethora of joy and pride.

This does not mean that you need to throw out all of your baby books or advice given by family and friends. What it means is you will use the books and advice as guidelines, but you also need to pay attention to your instincts. A mother's instinct is real and you need to use this to help modify the guidelines you are given so they are the best for your baby. You know what is best for your baby. Many times, us moms let the sleep deprivation take over, which makes us question every choice we make.

You will get a nonstop list of suggestions, tips, and hear, "you should try..." throughout the entire course of your child's life. It is not only impossible to utilize all this advice, it is also simply not what your baby needs. Trust your maternal instincts and tune out all the external chatter. You know what's best for your baby, and you just need to trust your own judgment.

The Process Is a Gradual One

No matter what method you use or when you start sleep training, it is a gradual process. You will need to have a lot of patience to get through sleep training, but you will become successful as long as you remain consistent. It is also important to note that you should not feel guilty when you are losing your patience. Instead, you need to take a moment to yourself. I remember one of my friends calling me the first night they started the sleep training process with their seven-month-old baby. I knew she needed help as I heard her little girl crying in the background and she told me, "You hear that? I have been listening to that for almost half an hour now. I have picked her up so many times until she calmed down. I place her back in her crib and I get this. I really want to sleep train, but I don't think I can do it. It's so hard. I just want to scream and cry with her."

I listened to her and I responded, "It is okay to go into another room and take a breather. Take a break, do your best to collect yourself, tell yourself 'I got this' and bring a little more patience into your system and try again. You will do this because you are a wonderful mom and you are giving your baby exactly what she needs." While she was hesitant, she decided to follow my advice. She called me back about 45 minutes later and she said, "She is finally asleep. After I calmed down a little bit, she calmed down a little. I still had to pick her up several times, but she is asleep. The first part of the night is over."

When you are calm, your baby will be calm. Remind yourself that your baby is safe, and in order for you to better help them, you need to take a few breaths. It is ok to take a break to collect yourself. This will benefit both you and your baby.

Key Points to Remember

- Every baby is different. There is no clear cut, one-size-fits-all effective way to sleep train.
- Do what works best for you and your family, which will take some adjustments by all those in the household.
- Trust your maternal instincts.
- Being consistent with the process will increase your likelihood

of success, even when things get worse or schedules are thrown off. Stay as consistent as possible.
- When you are calm, your baby will begin to calm down; take a few minutes when you need to gather yourself and be there for your baby. They tune into your energy more than you realize.

CHAPTER 6: Let's Get Sleeping, But First Thing's First – Safety

Before you take any steps into sleep training, you need to think about safety. Of course, this is something you always think of and several times a day, but you need to understand that safety plays an important factor in making their sleeping area safe. This means we need to discuss topics that mothers do not like to talk about—ones that just the thought of scares us to our core, such as Sudden Infant Death Syndrome (SIDS).

Please note: SIDS is not a topic we discuss to scare you or make you feel paranoid when your baby is sleeping, especially if they are sleeping in another room. It is here so you understand the topic and know what you can do to decrease the chances of SIDS. It is here to give you peace of mind. So, take a deep breath, and let's look at this together.

Whether you are a first-time parent or you just brought home your fourth child from the hospital a month ago, you are sleep deprived. You are practically begging your baby, partner, and other family members for just "a few more minutes." We always think we need "just a few more minutes." The problem is these few more minutes can become unsafe for your baby, yet you need to do what you can to get adequate sleep so you do not place your baby in an unsafe situation. At this point, you might be asking "What? Did she just say I shouldn't take the extra few minutes because they are unsafe, but to make sure I get good sleep?" Yes, I did; let me explain.

I have read news stories where parents heard their baby crying, yet they were so tired they could barely open their eyes. Spending the night at a friend's house years ago, I found her sleeping through her baby's cries because she was so tired. Here is one main fact about sleep deprivation: your body will make sure you get to sleep when you really need it. For some people, your body will put you in such a deep sleep that your screaming baby cannot wake you up. Yes, I understand the thought of this is frightening. For some of you, your partner or another child might get up to help your baby or wake you up. But, many of you do not have this option. My friend was a single mom and this was her first baby. To this day, we do not know if she slept through her baby's cries before or after I spent the night, but I do know that she did what she could to get better sleep so she could wake up for her baby. Because your body will put you into a deep sleep when you are sleep deprived, you need to do what you can to get the sleep you need as well.

There are many stories of sleep deprivation in mothers that have happy endings, but many do not. We all know the stories. I know of too many women whose babies passed away from SIDS over the last few years. One mother felt her baby was too cold without a blanket. It was one of the coldest nights of the year and she could not bear to lay her baby down without a blanket. She covered her baby up, laying the blanket near her baby's chest. When she went to check on her baby, the blanket had moved up toward the baby's mouth. Fortunately, it had not covered the baby's nose...yet. As you can imagine, this story could have a worse ending. Unfortunately, it does for some mothers.

Co-sleeping is a great feature if you support it. However, your baby can wake you up in the middle of the night with a thump as they bump their head into the wall or from screaming because they are stuck between the bed and the wall. Your blankets and pillows can cover your baby's face. There are many dangers when it comes to co-sleeping that you have to consider before you place your baby in your bed. One of my family members wanted to co-sleep with their baby because they felt this was the right choice to make. They did all the research they could about the subject and decided that setting a bassinet next to their bed was similar to co-sleeping and safer. One night she woke up to her baby's muffled cries as part of her blanket fell into the bassinet and covered the baby's face. She then switched her baby to their crib but set that next to her bed. While many would argue this is not co-sleeping, it was the safer option and this is what mattered.

The bottom line is, many safety mistakes happen because mothers are sleep deprived, they do not have the right information, or they think that "It will be okay." What you need to know about your baby's safety is extensive, so let's get to this information.

Sudden Infant Death Syndrome (SIDS)

While some babies will sleep better on their stomach than their back, this is not safe for your baby. Until your baby can lift up and turn their head on their own, you need to take all the safety precautions you can to ensure that your baby's sleeping area is suitable for them.

SIDS is the unexplained and sudden death of a baby under one year of age. Most deaths occur when a baby is between one and four months old. While researchers have searched for decades for the main cause of SIDS, there is no one answer. The only conclusions they have reached are the ways in which parents can decrease their chances of or prevent SIDS:

- **Blankets and pillows.** We are used to blankets and pillows and come to believe that we need them to keep warm during the night. We are comfortable with them and it is hard to sleep flat on our back without a pillow propping up our heads. Therefore, some parents automatically think that this is what their baby needs as well. They might have had a pillow and blanket as a baby and feel it is just what you do because it is what their parents did. But, blankets and pillows can quickly and easily become dangerous for your baby, especially when they are unable to move their head or move the object that is causing them to struggle to breathe. Leave blankets and pillows out of your baby's sleeping space until they can move their head or for a little longer.

- **Stuffed animals and other toys.** Stuffed animals and other toys are similar to blankets and pillows, especially stuffed animals. However, other kinds of toys also present another danger as many can be hard and have sharp edges for your baby. If they tip over in the crib, this could harm your baby. It is best to keep stuffed animals and toys away from your baby's sleeping space. This includes any toys that you can hang on the side of the crib, especially if your baby can reach them. Babies are tougher than we think and they can grab and pull on something tightly.
- **Car seats.** I have heard too many stories lately about babies falling asleep in their car seats and being left there only for their lips to be blue minutes later. It is always better to take your baby out of their car seat, even when they are sleeping well and try to lay them in their crib to continue sleeping. The biggest reason sleeping in a car seat is dangerous for a baby is because they have a little, heavy head that they cannot control or lift up. If their head falls forward too much, this can cause difficulty breathing and they can suffocate. I know you do not want to wake a sleeping baby, especially if they have not been sleeping, but safety is always first. The same goes for strollers or swings.
- **Check daycare policies.** None of us want to bring our baby to daycare, but many of us have no choice. You need to get back to work or you need someone to watch your baby because your

babysitter could not make it. Whether you are looking for a regular daycare provider or need someone ad hoc, you always want to make sure that your daycare provider considers your baby's safety. Ask about their policies and read through them like fine print. Interview them so you can get to know them. You can ask questions about car seats, sleeping arrangements, the type of help they receive from staff, etc. If you do not feel right about anything, even a single answer, then move on to the next person. Your instincts will always guide you as a mother.

- **No sleeping near windows or around strings.** Your baby moves more than you realize and the strings from the blinds can wrap around their neck. You should never have a pacifier connected to your baby because the string can become loose and cause your baby to suffocate or choke during the night.

According to the American Academy of Pediatrics, the main factors you should always remember when it comes to preventing SIDS are the following (American Academy of Pediatrics, n.d.):

- Until your baby turns one, they should share a bedroom with you, which is called room-sharing. They need to have their own safe sleeping space.
- Do not let anyone smoke, drink, or use drugs near your baby. If someone starts smoking when your baby is around, bring your baby to a healthier breathing environment.
- Lay your baby down to sleep in their sleeping space, which includes a firm mattress and a tightly fitted sheet.
- Ensure that your baby's crib is bare, other than their mattress and sheet. You should not have bumpers along their bed, blankets, pillows, stuffed animals, etc.

Back-to-Sleep Approach

It used to be normal for babies to sleep on their stomachs, and some babies will sleep better on their stomachs. However, the single most effective way that you can lower the chances of SIDS is by placing your baby on their back to sleep. If you feel that your baby will benefit from sleeping on their stomach, you need to discuss this with your baby's pediatrician. You should not place your baby on their stomach to sleep as they can fall into a deep sleep and not wake up when they need to move their head. This is one reason that you need to follow the back-to-sleep approach, which is having your baby sleep on their back. Another reason to follow this approach is some people believe laying your baby on their stomach can compress their diaphragm, which keeps them from getting the oxygen they need.

If your baby is struggling to sleep on their back, there are a few ways you can encourage back sleeping, which will give your baby a better chance of becoming comfortable:

- Lay your baby down when they are just about to fall asleep. They might be in a half-asleep and half-awake state, but they are too tired to wake up and notice how they are sleeping. If you are not sleep training and you have a newborn, you can lay them down when they are sleeping.
- Allow for plenty of tummy time when your baby is awake. Your baby needs to have their tummy time and they might be fighting to sleep on their back because they need this time.
- You can place a very thin pillow under your baby's mattress. This will help them prop them up a little bit without increasing their chance of SIDS. Babies feel more secure when they are curled a little bit as this is what they are used to, but placing them in a car seat, bouncer or stroller to nap is dangerous.

- Give your baby a pacifier, but make sure it is not connected to their clothing by a ribbon or string.
- Remain consistent. No, it is not fun to hear your baby cry and you want to do what you can to ease their troubles and make them comfortable, but their safety is always the number one priority. When you consistently lay your baby on their back, they will become used to sleeping this way.
- Do not worry if your baby starts rolling to their stomach during the night. They will start rolling around four to six months of age, and if they can roll over, their risk of SIDS has decreased significantly.

Safety With Co-Sleeping

It is important to note that co-sleeping and room-sharing are entirely different. When you co-sleep with your baby, they are in the same bed as you. You two are sharing a sleeping space. When you are room-sharing with your baby, you have their crib or bassinet in your bedroom, but you each have your own sleeping space. It does not matter where you set the crib, other than you want to make sure it is not near any windows, lamps, etc.

Parents enjoy co-sleeping because of the many advantages it offers:

- Both babies and parents get more sleep.
- If you nurse, it is easier to feed your baby when they are close to you without having to wake them. Usually, you will wake up when you start feeling your baby stirring, allowing you to start dream feeding them.
- You will limit your baby's nighttime separation anxiety, which usually starts between six to ten months of age.
- You will feel less stressed when it comes to laying your baby

down.
- You get to wake up to your baby looking, cooing, and smiling at you, which always helps make your day ten times better.

Co-sleeping is one of the biggest debates right now because people feel there is always a risk when it comes to placing your baby in your bed. Fortunately, there are many safety measures you can take when it comes to co-sleeping so both you and your baby feel safe and comfortable enough to get a good night's sleep.

First, before you think of bed-sharing, do your best to note how you fall asleep and how you wake up. Some people barely move when they are sleeping while others toss and turn most of the night. If you wake up and your blankets and pillows are out of order, you might want to rethink bed-sharing. When blankets and pillows move because you toss and turn, you run the risk of them moving closer to your baby.

If you have pets, try to make sure that they do not sleep in the bed with the baby. You also want to try to keep any other children from coming into the bed with you, which can start to stress younger children. For example, a young toddler will not understand why the baby can sleep with you but they cannot. In this case, you might want to try placing your baby's crib or bassinet close to your bed and allow your other child to sleep on the other side of the bed, so you are between your children. Most children move around a lot when they are sleeping, especially young toddlers.

You do not want to lay your baby down where they could get stuck between the bed and the wall or roll off the bed. Keep your baby's head away from any headboards so they do not bump their head during the night.

There are times where you should never co-sleep with your baby (Co-sleeping with your baby, n.d.):

- Your baby was born prematurely, before the 37th week.
- You or your partner smoke or have been drinking.
- You or your partner is a very deep sleeper.
- You are overtired.
- When your baby was born, they were less than five pounds.
- If you are sleeping on a sofa or an armchair. It is extremely dangerous to co-sleep in this way as it increases the risk of SIDS by 50%.

The point of this section is not to tell you that you should not co-sleep with your baby. If you feel that co-sleeping is the best option for you, your baby, and your family, then that is your choice to make. Let your instincts guide you. The purpose is to inform you of any safety measures you need to take so you can keep your baby safe.

Other Safety Tips

There are many safety tips that can be discussed, and while I would love to cover every one of them, there are just too many to fit in these pages. You will receive a plethora of tips and advice from other parents and non-parents alike. Here, I will try to give you as many of the useful and life-changing tips that I have gathered over the years. I know how much I treasured all the safety tips I received (and more have come out since then) and want to share this knowledge in hopes it is as helpful to you as it was to me:

1. If you feel so tired and are worried that there is a chance that you could fall asleep, do not sit in a rocker or chair while feeding your baby. If you can feed them while they lay in a bassinet next to you, great. If this is not an option, lay them in the bed by you.

When you wake up, place them back in their sleeping space right away. If you are worried about your blankets or pillows covering the baby, remove them until your baby is safely in their crib.
2. Change the positions your baby sleeps in as they are sleeping on their back. You can do this by gently moving their head into different positions, lay them in different places within their crib, or by moving the crib around the room so they become interested in looking at different parts of the room. The point is to keep their head from becoming flat on one side.
3. You can swaddle a newborn when they are about to sleep. This will keep them from waking up to their natural reflexes. If you do not swaddle them, as some babies do not care for it, then you want to have mittens on your baby's hands and keep their little nails trimmed and smooth so they do not cut themselves.
4. When your baby is awake, encourage them to have some "tummy time." This is when you can put a blanket on your floor and let them lay on their tummy. They will squirm, but you will also notice they are trying to lift up their head. This will make their neck muscles stronger and they will learn to move their head more and make you feel more at ease when it comes to their safety.
5. Ensure that no matter who is taking care of your baby, from a family member to a daycare provider, that they understand your safety measures and are willing to follow through.
6. Always check the temperature of your baby's room and your baby. You want your baby to be warm, but they can quickly overheat. The most comfortable sleeping temperature for your baby is between 65 and 72 degrees Fahrenheit or 18 to 22 degrees Celsius.
7. Do not dress your baby in clothing that does not fit them

properly. They need to be dressed in clothing that is snug but not too tight.
8. Do not have any type of electrical outlet or anything plugged in around your baby's sleeping area. Keep lamps and nightlights away from the bed and ensure all cords are not in reach of your child.
9. Always have a working smoke detector in your baby's room. Test the smoke detector often and change the battery at least every six months or when you hear the beeping warning that the battery is low.
10. It is normal for your baby's hands and feet to feel a little cold. This is not a good indicator of their body temperature. You want to look for signs of sweating or touch their stomach or back of the neck. If their tummy is warm, your baby is warm and you want to change their pajamas into something cooler or turn down the heat in their bedroom.

Key Points to Remember

- Reduce the risk of SIDS by keeping blankets, stuffed animals, and pillows out of your baby's crib.
- Be sure your baby's crib is kept away from strings and cords.
- Always double and triple check daycare centers or babysitter credentials.
- Always place your baby to sleep on their backs and give them plenty of tummy time during the day to reduce the struggle of back sleeping.
- Co-sleeping works for many parents but implement safety precautions. Room sharing can be a safer alternative.

CHAPTER 7: The Importance of Your Baby's Day and Nighttime Routine

Routines are important when it comes to your baby. The trouble is, especially for first-time parents, when it comes to routines, people normally think of a sleeping and feeding routine. The truth is, your baby's whole day should be taken into account, and a routine must be adhered to.

First, you need to remember every baby is different. You hear those wonderful stories mothers share that their baby started sleeping through the night by two months of age. You look at your little bundle of joy, who is three months old, and wonder why you are not that lucky. The fact is that some babies will be good sleepers from the time they are born while other babies will only sleep for a short period of time.

The best step you can take to help your baby get the amount of sleep they need is to educate yourself when it comes to routines and your baby's needs. We have already discussed healthy sleep, so you are on top of your research. Now, you are ready to dive into the importance of routines.

Benefits of Routines

- **Routines help your baby feel relaxed.** Children thrive when they are put on routines because they know what comes next. Routines help your babies feel secure and comfortable. They need this feeling so they can focus on learning throughout their day. Even when you think your baby is simply having tummy time and looking all over the room, they are doing so much more. They are learning about their environment. They know where you are and what you are doing. They notice anyone else in the room and what objects are around their environment.

- **Routines can help you relax as well.** It is not always easy to identify what your baby needs when they are crying. But when you get your baby used to a routine, you will know when they are telling you that they need a diaper change, need to eat, are tired, or need some attention. Knowing that your baby is fussy 45 minutes after they eat helps you note that it is time to change their diaper. This gives you an upper hand because you are not struggling to try to figure out why your baby is fussy or crying. Most parents automatically think that when their baby is crying, they are hungry, but this is not true. As you learned before, babies cry for many reasons. The best piece of advice is if you have recently fed your baby and they are crying, they are probably not hungry. Do not start reflectively feeding your baby just because they are crying. You need to look at the routine, listen to their cry, and try to figure out why they truly are crying.
- **Routines, especially a bedtime routine, help your baby sleep better.** You will see later how you can establish a calming bedtime routine to help your baby sleep. It is also important to note that a bedtime routine is not the only routine that will help your baby sleep better. When they are on a nap and feeding routine, they will sleep better as well. Ideally, their whole day should be scheduled.
- **Routines help babies during their transitional periods.** Because your baby is constantly developing, they go through a lot of transitional periods. These times are hard on your baby and can cause them to lose sleep because these periods are a bit stressful for them. The routines will give them security and help ensure they get the sleep they need.

Daily Schedules

When it comes to establishing a routine for your baby, you can do what you feel is best. The information discussed in this section is merely suggestions. You can use the following routines as a tip or a guide to creating your own. Remember, the best step for you to take is to follow your instincts. Do not second-guess yourself or think the experts or any other mother knows what is best for your baby. No one knows your baby better than you do. Therefore, if you feel that a bath isn't the best fit for your baby's nighttime schedule, but more of a way to help calm them before you allow them to play and tire themselves out a little more, then this is what you should do.

Daytime and Nighttime Feedings

When it comes to feeding your newborn during the day, you need to be more flexible. They will find their own routine and you need to follow through. For example, they might eat every three hours on the dot, such as 9:15 a.m., 12:15 p.m., and so on. You might also have a baby who tends to eat every two to three hours. Sometimes they will wait almost three hours for their next feeding and other times they can barely wait another two hours. A feeding schedule for your newborn might look like this:

- Breastfeeding on demand. You might feed them between seven to twelve times during a 24-hour period.
- You will also pump eight to ten times a day. You will not want to go for six hours (or more) without pumping.
- If your baby is on formula, they will eat about four to five ounces every feeding. They can feed about eight to ten times in a 24-hour period.

When your baby gets to be around four to five months of age, their schedule will start to shift as they will not feed as much during the day. When this happens, you can start to help them find their new routine. Because you will start introducing them to solid foods, such as adding rice in their milk, they will remain full for a longer period of time, especially during the night. Rice milk can help reduce your baby's feedings to one or two feeds a night.

Once your baby reaches the six-month mark, you can start putting them on a daytime feeding schedule a bit more. Six-month-olds who drink formula are now down to feed about four to five times a day. They are also drinking about six to eight ounces during each feeding. When it comes to breastfeeding, you are still following their demand when they are hungry. It is important to note that around six months of age is when you start introducing your baby to other solid, pureed foods. You might offer them a bottle and then set them in their high chair to eat a little baby food.

Between nine to twelve months, you can offer more solid foods, but you want to make sure that your baby cannot choke on the food. Also, make sure their food has all the nutrients your baby still needs and is in softer textures as their teeth are still coming in.

Around the one-year mark, your baby is starting to eat more with the family and this is becoming their routine. Of course, they will still have snacks and milk between their meals. If your family has specific dietary restrictions or preferences, you will need to discuss this with your baby's primary care doctor so you can make sure your baby gets all the nutrients necessary for their brain development and growth.

Nighttime Routine

Before you get settled into a nighttime routine, you want to be able to understand the cues your baby gives you when they are tired. For example, they might rub their eyes, stare into space, flick their ears with their fingers, become still and quiet, lose interest in their toys or people, or yawn and stretch often. You can figure out the sleepy cues your baby gives by observing them throughout the day. If you start to notice that it is a half-hour before you normally lay them down, start paying attention to their actions. If they are already giving off cues that they are tired, you might need to look at moving your child's bedtime forward. Of course, you will want to do this slowly. For instance, if you put them to bed around 7:30 p.m. and you see that they are giving you sleepy cues at 6:45 p.m., you want to aim to get them to bed at 7:00 p.m. Instead of jumping up and placing them in their crib, they will know that their schedule is off and become stressed or upset, you want to gradually move the time up by seven to ten minutes. For three days, you will get them to bed at 7:20 p.m, then you will change the time for 7:10 p.m., and then to 7:00 p.m. a few days later.

One of the best parts about a nighttime routine is that it is just you and your baby. You can bring a lot of quality time into the nighttime routine. While experts state that a nighttime routine should not last longer than 20 minutes, you need to focus on what is best for your baby. If your baby takes a bath for 15 minutes, you will probably not finish up the nighttime routine in 20 minutes. No matter how much time you spend on the routine, the main ingredients are consistency, patience, and love.

There is a lot of debate on how old your baby should be when you start a nighttime routine. Some people feel you should wait until they are three months old, while others feel you can start as young as five weeks old. Follow your baby's cues and what you feel is right. There is no right or wrong answer when it comes to starting a nighttime routine at a certain age. You can even sleep train your toddlers.

One of the cues I used to note when starting sleep training was my son's self-soothing techniques. Babies will naturally start to soothe themselves by folding their hands, coo, or put their finger in their mouth.

A suggested bedtime routine:

1. About 45 minutes before your baby falls asleep, give them a nice and warm bath. This will help make them feel calm and allow them to fall asleep easier. The trick is, especially when they become older, to keep them calm after their bath. This means you will not want to play any games that will get them running or too excited.
2. Quarter of an hour later, you can put their pajamas on and dim the lights in their room. If their room does not have a dimmer, you want to keep a lamp on or some type of low light instead of their main ceiling light.
3. 15 to 20 minutes before they fall asleep, you can give them a nightly feeding. There is a lot of debate about feeding your baby before bed. Some people say continuing to do this will result in your child becoming dependent on falling asleep only after a feeding. Other people feel that if you feed them right before they fall asleep, they will sleep for a longer period of time. Do what is right for you and your family.
4. After you burp your baby, find a calming activity, such as quietly singing a lullaby or reading a short story. I know people who spend a few minutes holding their baby in their arms and talking to them about the day. They would say positive statements such as how proud they were for what milestone(s) they accomplished that day or tell them what is changing in their life.
5. About five minutes before it is time for them to sleep, your baby

should be drowsy enough for you to lay them down. At this point, you need to follow your sleep training routine. This means if you need to caress their cheek as they fall asleep, you start doing this. If you are near the end of the sleep training period and you simply say goodnight and walk out of their room, you follow this procedure.

Nap Routine

The first factor you should know when it comes to naptime routines is the debate between parents and experts on whether it should closely follow your baby's bedtime routine or if it should be different. Some people believe they need to be different routines so your child understands when it is time to nap and when it is time to go to bed. While I understand this argument, I never notice any confusion with my child when I placed them down for a nap versus their bedtime. Instinctively, I felt that my baby would learn best by keeping the same routine, especially when I was sleep training him. Therefore, when I was at the point of standing next to his crib, rubbing his cheek as he tried to fall asleep, I did this whenever I put him to bed. Honestly, I feel that it helped him understand the process easier. It felt more consistent than only following the sleep training routine when he went to bed.

However, there are factors that you can change, especially as your child grows older. For example, if I would have read a book to my toddler before a nap like I did before I put him to bed for the night, he would sleep longer. I always had to wake him up from a nap if I read to him. If I did not read to him or I just made up a quick one to two-minute story, he would almost always wake up when he normally did. This was something I found out through trial and error—trust me, this is a part of parenthood.

When it comes to placing your child down for a nap, follow your instincts. If you feel it helps them to follow the bedtime routine, minus a bath if that is part of the routine, then this is what you do. Otherwise, you can devise a whole new routine to help your child sleep peacefully during their nap just like they do during the night.

When it comes to your newborns, until about the age of three months, you will need to go with the flow. You need to be flexible when it comes to schedules. Once your baby is around three to four months old, you can begin to incorporate a daily schedule into their day.

A daily schedule for a four- to five-month-old will depend on how many naps they are taking during the day.

If your baby is taking three naps during the day, their schedule may look like this:

- Your baby should wake up between 7:00 and 7:30 a.m.
- For their first nap of the day, you will lay them down at about 10:00 a.m. and allow them to sleep for an hour.
- You will want to lay your baby down at about 1:30 p.m. for their second nap. You will wake them up at about 3:30 p.m.
- You will lay them down for their third nap around 5:00 p.m. and allow them to sleep for about 30 minutes. You want to wake them up by 5:30, so they will have about two to two and a half hours before they go to bed.
- Bedtime should be between 7:30 and 8:00 p.m. They should sleep about 11 or more hours during the night, whether they are waking up for a few minutes or not.

For a baby at this age with two naps, their schedule may look like this:

- You should get your baby up for the day between 7:00 and 7:30 a.m.

- Your baby's first nap of the day should start at 10:00 a.m. and they should be awake by 11:30 a.m.
- You should lay your baby down for their second nap around 2:00 p.m., and they should sleep for two hours.
- Your baby's bedtime should be between 7:00 and 7:30 p.m. They should sleep for about 12 hours.

Your baby will follow a schedule similar to this until they are close to one year of age, which is normally when they will go down from two naps to one. Most pediatricians like children to continue their daily nap until they are about three years old, depending on your child. If your toddler is not tired when their bedtime rolls around, you will need to look into decreasing the amount of time they sleep during the day or talk to their doctor about stopping their naps.

Breaking the Nurse to Sleep Habit of Your Newborn

You love that moment. The moment where you are nursing your new, precious little one, the one who you longed to meet for nine months. Even when you are overtired, the moments that they look at you when they are nursing are moments you will never forget. Sometimes, you wish they can last forever but you know they cannot. You might feel it is important to break the nursing to sleep habit before you start sleep training. If you do, here are some tips to help you get through this time.

First, you want to understand that your baby will get hungry throughout the night. Therefore, one way to help them break the nursing habit is to feed your baby 15 to 20 minutes before they fall asleep. This way they are not dependent on your feeding to fall asleep and they will have a full tummy for several hours before they wake up because they are hungry. You can work this feeding into their nightly sleep routine. When it comes to weaning them off from nighttime feedings, this is one of the most effective ways to break the night waking cycle.

Dream feeding is another method that can be used to help transition baby into sleeping through the night. If you are considering starting to sleep train. you may find this dream feeding method useful. When you dream feed your baby, you feed them right before you go to bed between 10:00 p.m. and 12:00 a.m. You do not wake them up to feed them; instead, you will gently move your breast or the bottle toward your baby's bottom lip and move it back and forth slowly. Their natural eating reflex will catch on and they will start eating. Once they are done, and note they will not eat a regular amount, you lay them back down. Sometimes mothers note that their baby will wake up to eat again at 3:00 a.m., so they set their alarm for 2:45 a.m. and dream feed them again. It is always important to burp them after they dream feed. (Your baby will continue to sleep. You will always be amazed at what they can sleep through.)

Dream feeding is a step you can take when you are about to start sleep training and your baby is still feeding during the night because it allows them to get used to sleeping throughout the night for their age. Dream feeding, however, should be avoided when you actually begin to sleep train, as you want to teach your baby to fall asleep on their own when they are beginning to feel drowsy and not fall asleep as they are feeding. When sleep training, you want to stop feeding your baby when you notice they are beginning to doze off and lay them down so they can naturally fall asleep in their bed.

Cluster feeding is another way that you can help break the habit of nursing to sleep. This is when you will feed your little one often for a few hours before it is time for their nighttime routine. Cluster feeding is not the most popular way to help your baby wean nursing to sleep, but it works for some parents.

Key Points to Remember

- Routines benefit both you and your baby.
- Customize day and night routines to fit your baby's needs.
- While sleep training, you want to help wean your baby from the habit of waking to be fed or relying on being fed to get them to sleep. Before sleep training, you can utilize the dream feeding method, and then transition to the sleep training process and eliminate this method as you progress. Choose the method that works best for you.

CHAPTER 8: Ready, Set, Sleep

You always want to remember the main goal: to ensure your baby is sleeping comfortably in their bed so that they can fall asleep on their own and sleep well. The goal, though most people believe this, is not to get them to sleep through the night. To understand this, it is important to look at what sleeping through the night means—not waking up during the night. Not even for a minute. As an adult, you have done this many times (and you are probably craving another night like this) but babies do not sleep through the night. It is natural for a baby and the beginning stages of a toddler to wake up a few times throughout the night. Therefore, the main goal is to get your baby to self-soothe themselves back to sleep. When they wake up, they will only do so for a minute or two. In fact, they might not fully wake up. They will be in a half-asleep, half-awake setting.

Tips to Help You During the Sleep Training Process

1. **Remember to notice their signs of fatigue.** It might take you a few nights to notice your baby's cues to tell you that they are getting sleepy, but once you have identified these signs, you need to put your baby to sleep as soon as possible. It should be no later than 30 minutes from seeing these signs. Some of the signs they could give you are pulling their hair, pulling their ears, or any other signs that indicate tiredness.
2. **A sleeping ritual helps them understand day and night.** Your baby will start to distinguish day and night when they are a couple of months old. You can further help this by creating a different naptime and nighttime routine. For example, if you

give them a bath, put them in pajamas, read to them, and then lay them down for nighttime; you can sing them a song for their naptime routine. I found that keeping the same routine (minus the bath) worked best for us. Once again, find what works best for you and your baby.

3. **Always put your baby to bed at the same time every day and night.** It does not matter if you are laying them down for the night or a nap, you want to make your time consistent.
4. **Have patience.** Each of these phases will last several days. You will know when it is time to switch to the next phase when your little one does not protest as much as they are falling asleep and they fall asleep sooner.
5. **Signal the start of your baby's day.** When you wake your child up in the morning, you want to turn on their light and open their shades. You can also have a little morning ritual with them, such as telling them good morning, asking them how they slept, or starting by playing a fun little game with them to help make sure they are in good spirits for the rest of the day.
6. **Crying rages.** Crying rages will happen and they can make you feel stressed because it feels as though your baby is inconsolable. When they get into this type of crying attack, it is really hard for your baby to calm down. They need your help, and the best way to help is for you to remain calm. If you need to take a minute to yourself, it is important to do so. Enlist help from your partner or someone else in your home. If you are alone, do your best to find your patient and calm nature (you are a mom; you've got this). Hold your baby and help them calm down. Hug them and tell them that they are safe and that you are there for them. Do not move around the room, just stand there and hold your baby. Do not put them back in bed until they are calm.

7. **Do not alternate caregivers within one cycle.** A baby's single sleep cycle is at least 30 minutes of uninterrupted sleep. Whether you have a partner or someone else to help you through the sleep training process, you want to make sure that one person puts your baby to sleep each time. If you have a partner, you might decide to alternate nights or shifts, or one of you might take on the main job of sleep training. While some parents decide to sleep train together, you should not switch during the same sleeping cycle (at least 30 minutes of completed sleep). Remember, it is important for you to get enough sleep as well, so you should have a plan in place that allows for each of you to get the sleep you both need. Taking turns in shifts will help both partners get enough sleep through the process. If one of you is always putting your baby to sleep for the night, the other can take over if your baby wakes in the middle of the night or the morning shift. Remember, you want to ensure you baby has slept for one sleep cycle (at least 30 minutes) before the other parent takes over. If you are having a rather difficult night putting your baby to sleep, it is fine to ask someone else to try. This will not cause too much stress on your baby. You should also be aware that switching during a single cycle can cause your baby to resist your attempts the next time. But, they will quickly go back into their routine as long as you continue the process.
8. **Do not forget about sleep regressions.** There are many reasons your baby can go through sleep regressions. This might happen because they are going through a developmental stage, traveling, or they are not feeling well. The best step to take during these moments is to remain consistent and continue to have patience. Stay in the sleep training stage you are in and simply focus on what your baby needs.

Four Steps of the Sleep Process

Before we get into the four steps, it is important that you remember every baby is unique. They are their own person and they will handle the sleep process differently. Some babies will learn one step within a few days while other babies will take a week or more. This is fine. Your baby will learn the process in their time. The key to teaching your baby each step of the sleep process is consistency and patience.

Yes, these two ingredients are something that you lack from time to time. I have been there, too. You are so exhausted from such little sleep that you feel as though you have no energy left to place your little one in their bed, even though it is their bedtime. Plus, they are sleeping so well on top of you. If you move them, there is a strong possibility that you will wake them up and you will be up for a couple more hours when you could fall asleep right now with them in your bed. These feelings are normal, but you want to find the energy (you do have it, you are their mom) and place them in their bed because they will learn the steps of the sleep process quicker.

Step One: Befriend the Bed

Set a chair next to your baby's crib and lay them down. Place your hand on their head and gently caress your baby until they fall asleep. If your baby starts crying and you cannot console them with your caresses, pick them up and comfort them with hugs. Do not say anything, sing to them, or walk around. You want to stand there and comfort them until they are calm. Place them back in their crib. If they start crying again, even if it is before you set them in their crib, make sure you first set them down and then try to calm them without holding them first. Continue to rub their cheek or pat them on the head. You will repeat this process until your baby falls asleep. You can sit in the chair if you need a break from standing. Be careful not to fall asleep yourself. Once your baby is asleep, quietly walk out of the room. When they wake up during the night and need you, repeat this process after you take care of their needs, such as feeding or changing.

When your baby falls asleep without any crying or fussing for four to five days, you can start moving on to the next step. You might find that you can sit in the chair and not have your baby worry about not feeling your touch. You might also find that you can take a couple of steps away from their crib when they are still awake, though sleepy. The key is to make sure that they do not give you too much objection for a few days. They might whine or make a little cry, but they will not wait for your caress to soothe them.

Step Two: Weaning From Touch

In the second step, you want to make sure that they fall asleep without your touch. You will lay them down in their crib and sit in the chair. You should only caress them, without picking them up, if they start fussing. Once your baby calms down, stop contact and continue to sit in the chair next to them. If your baby starts crying or fussing again, repeat the process of calming them with your touch while they lay there. If they do not calm down from your touch, pick them up and hold them while standing at their crib, just like in step one. Once they are calm, place them back down and sit down, but do not touch them unless they become fussy.

Once you have nearly a week of hardly any rejections at bedtime, you can move on to step three.

Step Three: Attendance Test

In this step, you want to push your chair further back to the doorway of your baby's room but make sure you are in their sight. If they start crying or fussing, walk to their crib and repeat the process of step two. You might notice that your baby starts crying every time you sit in the chair. You might want to move the chair a little bit closer and see if this makes your baby a little calmer. Sometimes parents like to slowly push their chair closer to the doorway of the room. For example, you will have your chair about a foot or two away from your baby's crib the first couple of nights you perform this step. Then, you will move it back another couple of feet and continue this process until you are at their doorway. You will only move your chair back when your baby does not fuss that you did so.

You might start to notice that your baby hardly cries at all, but they fuss often. This is a good sign as it is telling you that they are getting used to their sleep training. Continue to follow this step until they barely make a sound for four to five nights. Then you can move on to the final step.

Step Four: Goodnight, Darling

In step four, you will lay your baby down in their bed, give them a kiss, and tell them goodnight and that you love them. You can say whatever you feel is best to give your baby the sense of comfort they need so that they know you are still there for them if they need you, and then walk out of their bedroom. Even if your baby starts crying before you leave the room, you want to continue this action, wait a few seconds and only then come back in.

To help your baby adjust to this step and officially learn to self-soothe themselves to sleep, you do not want to stand on the other side of the door. Your little one will know that you are there and they will continue to cry because they will want you inside the room.

If you hear your baby cry, wait to see if they continue to cry before you rush in. You might tell yourself to wait 30 seconds to a minute before heading to the bedroom. The truth about your baby's little fuss or cry is that they can still be sleeping and rushing into the bedroom will wake them up.

Daytime Sleep

You will perform daytime sleeping in the same way as you will nighttime sleep. Even if your baby wakes up a half an hour early, you want to put them back to sleep so they can finish their nap. If it is getting close to their naptime and you notice that your baby does not show signs of tiredness, you want to start the ritual when you are supposed to as this will help make them tired.

Most babies tend to protest their naps a little more than bedtime. If you are struggling to have your baby take their nap because they are crying too much, you can try to lay them in another spot in your house to see if they will fall asleep. If they totally skip their daytime nap (it happens), then you want to make sure they get to bed a little earlier so they still get their daily sleep.

Night Feedings

To help control night feedings, you want to organize the feedings into no more often than once every three hours. You also need to ensure that your baby does not fall asleep when they are eating. Once you start to notice that their sucking is slowing down, you want to stop feeding them, even if they have not eaten very much (as babies do not tend to eat the same amount during the nightly feedings). If your baby wakes up before it is time for their nightly feeding, put them back to sleep by following your night training phase.

If you are struggling to get them back to sleep and it is coming close to their feeding time, you still want to ensure your baby falls back to sleep for at least 30 minutes before you feed them. You want your baby to enter into a sleep cycle, which is at least 30 minutes; if they wake before this time, you want to focus on getting them back to sleep before feeding. If your baby wakes up after they have slept for at least a half-hour, then feed them.

Key Points to Remember

- Every baby is different and it is important that you come up with a routine that is right for your baby and family.
- Consistency is key in order to be successful with sleep training. Some steps may take a day or two to achieve; others may take a few weeks. Be consistent with your efforts.
- The sleep training process consists of four easy-to-follow steps:
    1. Caress your baby to sleep.
    2. Sit next to your baby's crib until they are asleep.
    3. Gradually move the chair further away from the crib until your baby falls asleep.
    4. Kiss your baby goodnight and leave the room so your baby can fall asleep on their own.

CHAPTER 9: Sleep Regression and Problem Solving

Your baby is always growing and developing. It does not matter if you are looking at their physical, emotional, or psychological development. Keep in mind that even if you do not think your baby is learning certain skills from you, they will prove their knowledge down the road. For example, they will learn self-soothing techniques almost naturally as a newborn. These techniques will become important to them throughout their life, such as when they are learning to soothe themselves to sleep. Sleep regression may make you feel like you are going backward with your child's sleeping patterns. Understand that sleep regression is a normal process in your baby's development, and when they do occur, it is important to remain consistent with the sleep routines you have already established.

Sleep Regression: It Is Real

Sleep regression may feel like it lasts an eternity, but rest assured, this is just a phase. For most babies, this can last anywhere from one to four weeks. It is a period of time where your baby, who has been sleeping well and often through the night, will suddenly start to wake up during the night. They might wake up once, twice, or several times. Sleep regression often catches you off guard, which can be frustrating because you are now back to waking up during the night with your little one trying to coax them back to sleep.

Sleep regression occurs for many reasons. Your baby may be teething, sick, or hitting a major developmental milestone. You can prepare yourself for sleep regression by knowing when they will strike, what can trigger them, and the best ways to handle them at each age.

4-Month Sleep Regression

If your baby is not sleep trained by the time they are four months old, then you may not notice the sleep regression. This stage happens because they are losing their newborn sleeping patterns and following an adult pattern. They understand day and night a little better and are ready for longer, nighttime sleep. They may still be waking frequently throughout the night and may be taking short but frequent daytime naps.

Keep in mind that this is also a significant time in their development. Your baby is making plenty of outside connections with the world around them and their brain is filtering and organizing all this new information at an alarming rate. This is also a time that your baby goes through growth spurts that can interfere with their typical sleep patterns.

The four-month sleep regression period is often the hardest to overcome, so rest assured that when it occurs in the future, you will be better equipped to handle them. The most common signs that you are entering the sleep regression period at four months include:

- Your baby is fussier than usual.
- Your baby will wake more frequently at night.
- Your baby may not be napping as much or as long during the day.
- Your baby may not be eating as they usually would, either not eating as often or needing to eat more.

The four-month sleep regression period can last from two to four weeks. It is important that you remain calm as you and your baby will both be frustrated and suffering through this time together. Your baby is trying to learn and adjust to their own rapid growth and you are trying to soothe and comfort them the best you can. You can still encourage healthy sleeping habits during a sleep regression period and this can be a great time to assist your baby in learning and utilizing the new skills they are learning.

When sleep regression occurs, first ensure that your baby is not sick. If your baby is healthy and just not sleeping, there are a few things you can do to help promote longer nighttime sleep sessions:

1. **Encourage your baby to practice their new skills during the day.** It is not uncommon for babies who are learning to master a new activity like rolling over or sitting up on their own to wake in the middle of the night to practice. Just imagine how excited you would be if one day you would discover you could fly. Wouldn't you want to practice and enjoy your new skill day and night? This is exactly how your baby feels. Allow your baby to practice these new skills during the day by setting aside plenty of time for them to roll and sit as much as they like without interruptions.
2. **Refrain from nighttime feedings.** If your baby was sleeping through the night and they start to wake again, you might quickly think they need to be fed. If you revert back to nighttime feedings, you will have to restart the sleep training process to get them out of this routine again. Feeding them when they wake in the middle of the night will strengthen their association with being fed when they wake up. Instead, feed them enough during the day. When you are feeding them during the day, be sure it is done in a place that is designated for eating. This way your baby will not get distracted and will know this is the time

and place to eat. Also, feed them a little more just before they are about to sleep. When they have a full belly before bed, they will be less likely to wake up in the middle of the night hungry.

3. **Be sure their sleep environment is dark and encourages sleep.** Even during nap times, the room you have them sleeping in should be dark as this will help them make the connection at night that it is time to sleep. Keeping the room dark will also help them fall back to sleep quickly if they do wake up in the middle of the night. When they wake up in the morning, be sure to open the curtains or blinds and allow the natural light to fill the room. This will help them better distinguish between night and day and, therefore, will reinforce when they are supposed to be sleeping.

4. **Stick with your routine.** Set up napping schedules so that your baby is getting enough sleep each day. Be consistent with your routine, especially your nighttime routines.

5. **If your baby does wake in the middle of the night, allow them a few minutes to try to fall back asleep on their own.** If they continue to cry, check if they need to be changed. When you are changing their diapers in the middle of the night, try to do so as quickly and quietly as possible. Try to avoid turning on any light in the room so your baby does not become stimulated, which will cause them to stay awake for longer. When you are done changing their diapers, lay them back in their crib and encourage them to fall back asleep.

8- or 10-Month Sleep Regression

The next time you will typically encounter sleep regression is when your baby is between eight and ten months old. During this time, you may have been struggling to get your baby into a sleep routine and then the regression hits and you didn't think the terrible sleeping patterns could get much worse. Or your baby may have been sleeping soundly for a few months and then all of a sudden you are wondering where your amazing sleeping baby has gone and dread they might not come back. Whether you have been struggling with getting your baby to sleep or know how peaceful the nights can be when they do sleep, the 8- or 10-month sleep regression is not fun for any parent. Luckily, there are a number of ways you can get through this phase and get back to those peaceful nights.

Sleep regression at this age is often due to physical and mental developments and also because of the transition to fewer daytime naps. At this age, your baby may be moving more, whether sitting up on their own or attempting to crawl. This increase in movement means your baby is using up a lot more energy and moving their body in different ways they haven't been able to before. These new motor skills can be hard to resist, which means they will be practicing at every chance they get, often when they are supposed to be sleeping. While you would expect all this increase in activity to tire your baby out, they can quickly become overtired and so begins the vicious cycle of being too tired to sleep.

At this age, your baby is also able to recognize a lot more things in their surroundings. They are probably learning to make new sounds with their mouths, learning different colors, animals, and shapes. They are beginning to categorize things and are becoming more curious about how things taste, feel, look, and smell. During these months, your baby begins to grasp the concept of understanding that just because they cannot see something doesn't mean it is not still there; peek-a-boo is a favored game at this age. This understanding helps ease the separation anxiety your child may have struggled with in the past that caused you to have a difficult time putting your little one to bed.

Your baby is also gaining a better understanding of cause and effect. They may begin to test your limits with this new understanding by screaming forcefully for you to swoop in to meet their needs even when they may not necessarily need anything. How you respond and react to your child's behavior will determine whether this new behavior will become a habit or not.

The nap transition will also cause disruption to the evening routine. At this time, it is likely that your baby will be ready to go from three to two naps a day. You can tell when your baby begins to fight you on the late midday nap that their nap time or number of naps need to decrease. The other two naps will often decrease in length as well. This time will be made up for in the evening hours of sleep, but for the first week or two, you will be struggling with getting your baby used to these transitions. Your baby will be overly tired more often, and this is where the following tips should help reduce the stress that comes from a fussy little one who needs more sleep but fights you on it every step of the way.

Tips for the 8- or 10-month regression:

1. If your baby was having difficulty sleeping prior to the eight-month regression, there are additional sleep issues that need to be resolved first. If a routine has yet to be established, now is the time to commit to one. Pay attention to what your baby associates with sleep. At this age, they may have formed the wrong day and nighttime associations or may associate riding in the car with sleep. If you notice your little one always snoozing through an activity or at a certain time, you want to make any necessary adjustments and provide reinforcements that help them form the right sleep pattern.
2. Give your baby extra support with snuggles, attention, and

reassurance as you work together through the transition. If separation anxiety is still an issue at bedtime, give them some extra time to cuddle with you but lay them down when they are awake but drowsy.
3. Set structured times. Give your baby a lot of extra time during the day to work with them and let them practice all the new skills they are learning, such as crawling and standing.
4. Set an earlier bedtime. Since your baby will be taking fewer naps, you want to try to get them to sleep earlier than they typically would when they took three naps a day. This bedtime can be as early as 5:30 or 6:00 p.m. most nights, until they have fully adjusted to two naps a day.
5. Do your best to be aware of any new habits your baby may be forming around bedtime, and refrain from falling back into old habits. This regression phase will be short-lived; the habits they form will often be long term. You don't want to revert back to waking in the middle of the night feeding your baby or have to rock them back to sleep every time they wake. You also don't want to have to pick things up off the floor they keep throwing out just to get you back into the room (I'm personally guilty for letting this one happen.)

11- or 12-Month Sleep Regression

Not every family will encounter the 12-month sleep regression period, but many do. Sleep regression at this age is often due to the fact that many children are learning to walk and talk around this time. It can also take on a variety of forms. Your little one sleeps through the night but may now have trouble getting to sleep or may wake up after only sleeping for a very short period. Your once easy-to-place-in-their-crib-and-soothe-themselves to sleep baby may begin to scream and cry every time you try to place them in their crib. It is not uncommon for these occurrences to happen once in a while, but you'll know you are in a sleep regression when it occurs more often than not.

Many factors can contribute to sleep regression:

- Your baby is strengthening their awareness. You may notice that your little one is more interested in stacking things, opening and closing books, or lining things up. This increase in awareness is keeping them busy and curious. For them, figuring out all the things around them is much more interesting than sleeping, which is where the sleep regression comes into play.
- Some children begin to walk or talk, and sometimes both, around their first birthday. Even if your baby isn't walking or talking, there's a good chance they are moving about, be it crawling or holding onto the furniture around them. They may also be making many sounds and can at least identify their mom and dad. What is important to remember is that at this age, your little one may not be able to communicate fully with you just yet, but they understand a great deal more than you realize. Combine their new movement skills along with their talking skills and then add in the fine motor skills, there are a lot of exciting things your baby wants to perfect doing. Sleep isn't on the top of their interest list.
- When your baby reaches the one-year mark, there will once again be a change to their napping and sleep needs. At this age, your baby may still be sticking with two naps a day but they are probably fairly short in length. Some children may even be transitioning to just one nap a day once they are around 14 months old.

Sleep regression at this age can last up to six weeks. With proper planning and understanding of what is triggering your baby's sleep disturbance, you can help guide your baby back to healthy sleeping patterns. If you are going through a sleep regression with your little one, give some of these tips a try:

1. **Many babies at this age can have a lot of stored-up energy if they haven't had the opportunity to burn it off during the day.** An increase in daytime activities can help your baby sleep better at night. You want your little one to practice their walking, talking, and motor skills as much as possible during the day so they won't be enticed to do so when they are in their crib and supposed to be sleeping. Give your baby time to interact and play with different toys and try to avoid keeping them in the car seat or stroller for long periods of time. This will ensure that they are getting plenty of movement and opportunities to explore the world around them.

2. **Keep naps to two a day**. Your baby may be fighting with you during one of their daytime naps, which is a good sign that your baby is ready to transition to one nap a day. If your baby is not 14 months old, there is a good chance they are not ready for just one nap a day even if they are fighting you on it. The fighting you are encountering can easily be a result of the sleep regression at this time, so you want to avoid dropping one of the daytime naps until the regression has passed. Even if these naps are quite short or your baby is just spending some quiet time in their crib, they still need this rest or relaxation time. Wait until your baby is at least 14 months old before you start eliminating one of the daytime naps.

3. **Stay consistent.** It can be a struggle to get your baby to sleep during this regression but you want to keep up with the sleep schedule or routine you already have in place. Try not to

deviate from it as tempting as it might be. Your baby will adjust much better and be able to fall back into their routine when they know what to expect.

18-Month Sleep Regression

The 18-month sleep regression can be an exhausting experience. Your little one is about to enter into their toddler years and is full of personality. You may have thought that you have finally gotten the hang of their sleep schedule routine and then the regression hits and it's like you are back at the starting line all over again. Rest assured, as with any other sleep regression you have gotten through, this too shall pass.

Sleep regression at this age is most likely due to a growth or developmental spurt your child is going through. At the 18-month mark, your baby's brain is undergoing some rapid changes and this can cause those wonderful sleep-regulating hormones to get temporarily thrown out of balance. You might find you perfect little sleeper resisting rest, waking up multiple times in the night, or waking up and not being able to fall back asleep. If your child is not sick, teething, or adjusting to major external factors like travel or family stress, it is normal for your baby to go through this 18-month sleep regression.

While the 18-month sleep regression can be a frustrating experience, there are some ways you can help your child sleep more easily while staying calm during this time.

How to handle the 18-month sleep regression:

1. **Consistency should be the main focus of getting through the 18-month sleep regression.** At this point, since your baby's brain is going through so many changes, you need to

continually reinforce healthy sleep habits. Your baby's brain will need to be somewhat reprogrammed for sleep. At this time, it can be difficult for your little one to recall what they are supposed to do when they wake up in the middle of the night and they will need to be redirected and reminded that specific times are meant for sleep and not for playing or practicing newly acquired skills.

2. **Add in additional bedtime and sleeping cues for your child.** Your baby may be slightly overwhelmed by all the new changes their brain and little body is going through. Gentle, yet direct, reminders that bedtime is approaching can help them feel more at ease and be prepared for what is coming. Ensure that you have an established sleeping routine for naps and bedtime. The more predictable and simple this routine is, the easier it will be for your baby to transition into sleep mode.

3. **Provide comfort for your child but stick with the routine**. You want to remain calm during the 18-month sleep regression as your child will most likely be persistent with their efforts to stay awake longer. It is important that you set clear guidelines and boundaries for bedtime. You want to comfort your child at this time but also make it known that sleep is just as important as all the other activities your child takes part in during the day.

4. **Avoid short-term solutions.** During any regression, you want to avoid implementing any new solution that can have long-term effects. At this age, many parents might allow their children to sleep in the same bedroom when they wake up in the middle of the night instead of fighting with them and sending them back to their own room to sleep. They might also provide a night light for their child to use when they wake up in the middle of the night so they can quietly look at books or play while everyone else in the house is awake. While these

solutions, along with many others, may work for some families, for many others, this can result in them becoming new bedtime habits that you will then need to address later on. If the solution for waking up in the middle of the night is to sleep on the floor next to the parents' bed, understand this may be continued for many months even after the sleep regression has passed. If the solution you use for nighttime wakings is not something you would want to have to continue within the long term, you want to avoid using it as a solution. Stick with strategies that you will want your child to be able to use in the long term, and this will lead to more healthy sleeping patterns as they grow.

5. **At this age, your little one is probably exposed to a variety of screens**. They probably have a favorite show or like to watch YouTube videos or play educational games on a tablet. Technology can be a great tool that helps your baby learn and develop but screen time should be limited. There have been various studies that link sleep disturbance with excessive screen time. Each child is different; for some watching a few hours of television a day will have little to no impact on their sleep. For many others, watching just a short amount of TV can keep them up all night. As a general rule of thumb, you want to cut out screen time at least two hours before bedtime. The light from the television triggers brain activity and can keep your baby up for hours. Instead of screen time, use this time to do quiet activities like coloring, reading, building puzzles, or playing a game together. Not only will this give you extra bonding time with your little one, it will also get them into the habit of finding other ways to entertain themselves.

While the 18-month sleep regression is perfectly normal for children to go through, it can be concerning for parents. Sometimes all the strategies, consistency, and routines seem to have no impact on your baby sleeping through the night. This results in your baby not getting the proper amount of sleep, which can have long-term effects on their development. If your baby's sleeping patterns are a concern, here are some things to keep in mind, consider, and/or give a try:

1. **Consult a sleep professional.** There are plenty of sleep specialists that can assist you in helping your child learn the right sleeping skills they need. A professional might be able to provide you with additional strategies to use to help get your little one to sleep and to ensure that they are getting the right amount of sleep.
2. **Know the difference between sleep disturbances and sleep disorders.** Sleep disturbances are often temporary factors that can throw off your child's typical sleeping patterns. The trigger for these disturbances can often be identified as environmental factors or because of parental behaviors. If you have traveled recently, moved, or had visitors for a short while, these can cause your child to sleep less. If one or both parents exhibit stressful behavior, chances are that your child will often be able to pick up on this stress, which then causes them to feel uncomfortable when trying to sleep.
3. Sleep disorders, on the other hand, can often present additional concerns for parents. Many children who are suffering from a sleep disorder at this time can exhibit drastic behavior or physical changes. These are not always easy to identify as your child may be having behavior trouble due to the lack of sleep because of sleep regression. Since it can be difficult to determine if your child's behavior is just the result of a bad night's sleep or because of several nighttime interruptions, it is recommended that you call your child's doctor if you notice

your baby is sleeping significantly less than the recommended 12 hours.

4. **Understand that some medical conditions will often have a major impact on sleep.** Children who have special needs or those with psychiatric or developmental disorders will struggle more with sleep. If your child does have a diagnosis that impairs their sleep, learn how you can better establish healthy sleeping patterns for your child.

2-Year Sleep Regression

Just when you think you have gone through all the fighting and struggling, you get hit with the two-year sleep regression. Your baby is now a toddler and you are thinking that the "terrible twos" are sometimes an understatement when it comes to the fights that occur around bedtime. It feels like each night is a never-ending chore. First, they are thirsty, then too cold, then their pajamas don't feel right, then they are too hot, they need to use the bathroom, and more water, and so on. It can feel like no matter what you do to get your child to bed, they have a hundred other things that need to be done instead.

The two-year sleep regression is one that will test your sanity and patience. You will find yourself giving in to all the demands and needs of your little one just to get them to sleep because you yourself are exhausted and just want to get to bed. You will find yourself frustrated and fed up a number of nights and you will be implementing every single technique, tip, tool, and anything else that gives you hope of a full night's sleep.

First, during the dreaded two-year sleep regression, know that almost every parent goes through this battle. Many parents cave and just let their child do whatever they want just so that they can sleep, and at times, you will most likely cave too. Don't beat yourself up for it; every once in a while, you have to wave the white flag so that you can properly take care of yourself as well. Just know that when you wave the white flag, get the rest you need, so you can be better prepared for the next night's battle.

While this doesn't sound like much fun, there are some ways you can get through the two-year sleep regression with more sanity and success. There can be a number of reasons why your little one is putting up such a fight at bedtime all of a sudden. Often, when you can identify what is triggering the unwelcomed behavior at bedtime, you can better address the issue to avoid any prolonged bedtime struggles. Some of the most common factors that contribute to the two-year sleep regression can include:

- **Believe it or not, anxiety can be the number one cause that keeps your little one awake and fearing bedtime.** At this age, many children begin to develop fears when it comes to night time. Sometimes they are afraid of the shadows in their room, most often it is that they want their parents closer to them. When you are in the throes of a bedtime battle, stop and ask your child what might really be causing the struggles at night. Many of these are easy fixes: having a nightlight in their room, cuddling a little extra with mom or dad, or writing a special note for them to look at if they wake up in the middle of the night, that reassures them they are safe and that you are not that far away. The main step for addressing these types of anxieties is to reassure your child that you hear and understand their needs and fears. Many times, just acknowledging and talking about what can be causing their evening anxiety is enough to put a stop to it.
- **Transitioning to a toddler bed.** If you are considering moving

your child to a "big kid" bed or have already done so, this can contribute to the sleep regression. Now that they are more easily able to just get out of bed, they will be more tempted to do so and play instead of sleeping. Many cribs allow for you to lower the setting and move the mattress to the floor with the crib bars enclosing the mattress. Your child may be too big or your crib may not lower enough to keep them from climbing out. Toddler beds can provide your child with a safer sleeping space at this age, but you will need to set specific rules and follow through with them when the adjustments are made.

You will need to be extra encouraging when switching to a toddler bed. Getting your child to stay in bed will be the biggest accomplishment. This will take some time and you will need to check on them regularly. When they have stayed in bed each time you check on them, you want to praise them and point out how well they did with controlling themselves. You will need to implement excuses for you to leave the room and then come back a few minutes later to check on them. Once your child is able to remain in the bed, you want to build their confidence and congratulate them. They will begin to realize they are capable of successfully staying in bed without being frightened or scared. Since you have been checking in on them, they know that eventually you will return and this thought alone can help ease them to sleep.

- **Sleep regression can almost always be expected when a new baby arrives.** The new baby is now getting all the attention your child was used to getting and many of your child's things now have to be shared with their new sibling(s). This can be very upsetting for your child. They will want to have extra attention and will constantly be seeking out ways to have the same connection with you as they did before the baby came along. Many times, this will be in the middle of the night.

To help your little one cope with the new addition, you will want to acknowledge and address their behavior. This is best done through a playful activity like having them pretend they are the new baby. Your child will most likely let you know they are feeling ignored or that they wish they could spend more time with you doing something specific. You can also try a role reversal activity where your little one can pretend to be you at bedtime and you get to be them. Each of these activities should be done during the day hours and not actually in the evening before bed. This will allow you to work together to come up with an appropriate solution for the bedtime sleep routine.

- **A common issue that tends to occur during this regression is that your child will begin to wake up earlier than you'd like.** Your child may be sleeping the right number of hours but that tends to mean if you are still putting your child to bed at 6 p.m. they will be up around 6 a.m. It might be time to bump back their evening bedtime by an hour or two if you want them to sleep in a little longer in the morning. You can also utilize an alarm clock and explain to your child that when the clock reads a certain time, they can leave their rooms.
- **Resist the cry-it-out method.** While this method of sleep training may have been effective for some parents when their child was a baby (even though it is not generally recommended), many parents who try to utilize this method once their child is a toddler often see this escalate the frustrations. Using this method can also have a serious negative impact on your relationship with your child. This is the stage where you want to acknowledge and listen to your child's

needs, not ignore and let them soothe themselves. At this age, you will be working hard with your little one in trying to help them manage their emotions and begin to problem-solve for themselves. This regression period is ideal for working on both these vital skill sets. Instead of the cry-it-out method, which can result in behaviors that carry over to the day time activities, excuse yourself from the room and check back in on them.

- **Naps will be a struggle as well.** Some toddlers may be able to cut out their naps completely at this age, but most will still need that nap to relax and calm down. Even if your child does not nap every day, you still want to schedule in quiet, awake time that will allow your child to give their brains a break and rest. You don't want to keep them busy during this time as this can result in an overtired child in the evening, which, of course, will lead to a long battle to get them to fall asleep.

Whether you are thinking of cutting out their daytime naps or want to include them still, you will need to look at what time they are waking up in the morning. If your child is waking up early in the morning, and this works for you, you might want to include an early midday nap. If your child is waking up a little later, you might want to cut back the length of the nap from two hours to just one. Whichever nap schedule you choose, you want to be sure it is one you can stick with and be consistent with.

- **If you are struggling with your child waking up regularly in the middle of the night, this can be exhausting for parents.** Most children who wake in the middle of the night are unable to fall back to sleep unless all of their sudden needs are fulfilled. Many times, children will wake for some basic needs. Their room may be too hot or too cold, they may be getting sick or are in some kind of pain (growing or other), or you may need to look at what they are eating during the day. Many children at this age wake in the middle of the night because they are hungry. If your child's diet has many sugars, processed foods, or food additives, these can severely disrupt your child's ability to fall asleep and stay asleep. You want to ensure that your child's diet is filled with nutrient-dense foods that will keep them full and fueled during the day and allow them to rest at night.

- **Understanding bedtime fights.** When your little puts up a struggle every time they are put to bed, this is often due to two main factors. Either they want to be in more control of the situation or they are acting out in order to connect with you. When your child hits the two-year mark, it is inevitable that throughout the day they are expected to listen, follow directions, and do as they are told. When this is coming from the parents most of the day, your child will simply feel disconnected from you.

Children at this age are also likely to start wanting to have a little more independence and be able to make choices on their own. When this is taken away from them regularly during the day, you can guarantee you will be met with a power struggle at bedtime. One way you can help encourage your child's independence, strengthen your connection, and get them to comply with a bedtime routine is to create visuals for them to follow along with. You and your child can create the visuals together for extra bonding time, but do allow for your child to make some of the decisions as to what order they will do things and what appropriate bedtime activities they can do to help them relax and drift to sleep. The visuals also help you redirect your child when they become distracted or want to deviate from the agreed-upon routine.

Sleep regression in two-year-olds also has a lot to do with their brain development at this time. Your little toddler is beginning to experience a wide range of emotions that drive a number of their behaviors and choices. While not always ideal, your child may be acting out at bedtime because they need help coping with big emotions. When your child is tired, you can expect to see emotions accelerated. Your child needs your help to guide them through these emotions and to learn the appropriate way to express their feelings and resolve issues on their own.

Consistency Is the Key

I have said this so many times throughout this book because I really cannot say it enough: consistency is key. Of course, there are a lot of other pieces to the puzzle that are important, such as patience. But without consistency, the system will fail. Your baby learns through routine and you need to ensure that routines are consistent as this will help them learn the rest. Being consistent with the sleep routines will teach your child what to expect and what behaviors are acceptable at this time.

Sleep regression can be a challenging obstacle for you and your baby no matter what age it occurs at. But consistency is what will help both of you get through the struggle with more patience and less frustration. When sleep regression strikes, have a consistent routine in place for bedtime and naps. The key elements you should be consistent with include:

- **Having bedtime activities.** These activities might include having a small healthy snack, a bath, reading a book, cuddles,

then a good night kiss or hug.
- **Being consistent with how you will handle the middle of the night wake-ups.** Avoid reverting back to old solutions when your child wakes up in the middle of the night.
- **Setting bedtime boundaries and rules.** Go over these rules regularly through pretend play during the day when you hit a sleep regression period.
- **Giving your child plenty of time to play and exert their energy throughout the day.** Your child is learning many new skills and is eager to use them. Giving them the time throughout the day will help them resist the urge to use these skills when they are supposed to be sleeping.
- **Listening to what your child is saying to you.** Demanding your child to go back to sleep is not the ideal way to get your child to sleep better. Instead, try to understand what can be causing them to all of a sudden struggle with sleep and then work together to resolve the problem.
- **Ensuring their sleep environment is ideal for sleep.** Keep the lights off or at least low, keep the temperature around 68 degrees Fahrenheit, and ensure your child is safe in their crib or bed.
- **Cutting out screen time two hours before bedtime.** Encourage your child to do a quiet activity instead.

Key Points to Remember

- Sleep regression is a part of your child's natural growth systems.
- Sleep regression will commonly occur at 4 months, 8 or 10 months, 12 months, 18 months, and 2 years of age.
- Sleep regression is most often due to developmental progress,

your child's desire to connect more with you, or struggles with unfamiliar emotions.
- When sleep regression hits, consistency is crucial to getting through it and quickly returning to a healthy sleep schedule.

CHAPTER 10: Baby Is Sleeping but Are You?

As a mother, sleep is not the easiest part of your life, but it is not a luxury that you can take "when you get a moment." You need sleep in order to function your best. You need sleep so you can care for your baby. You need sleep because you need to take care of yourself. As a mother, having a baby who constantly wakes in the middle of the night is only one component of why you may not be getting enough sleep. Addressing the other causes for your lack of sleep can help you work through them and this will often result in you not feeling guilty about asking someone else to step in and take over while you catch up on sleep.

It can be challenging to handle a little one and a plate full of other responsibilities you have to tend to. You may feel guilty or undeserving of getting the rest you desperately need. But you deserve to be rested for yourself and your baby (and the rest of your family). While each parent is different, many moms struggle through the same issues when it comes to skipping out on their own sleep routine, and we will address the most common ones so you can set up a consistent sleep routine for yourself as well.

Sleeping Problems of a Young Mother

It seems as though it is normal for many moms with children under six months old to get an average of three hours of sleep a night, with many nights only equating to an hour of uninterrupted sleep. While losing a few hours of sleep when your new baby comes home is expected, taking on a six-month-long sleep-deprived responsibility is not ideal or healthy. Moms are undoubtedly some of the most sleep-deprived individuals in the world. What is alarming is that while moms are getting little to no sleep night after night, often they are the ones responsible for caring for the baby for most of the day on their own. Why, then, is sleep not a more important factor?

Sleep problems in young mothers can actually begin prior to your baby being born. How many times did you have to wake in the middle of the night for something? How many nights did you simply roll back and forth trying to find a comfortable position? How many times did restless leg syndrome, backaches, nausea, or any other ailment keep you from getting good quality sleep? If you were lucky enough not to struggle with any of these issues, you may have suffered through more emotional or mental blocks. You may have found yourself up late at night worrying about how healthy your baby will be, or if you will make the right choices for them, or do you have enough diapers for when they arrive? Or maybe you just kept running over what you have packed in your hospital bag for when the arrival day comes. Chances are you were already training yourself for the sleepless nights that were to come once your little one entered the world. For many mothers, this is the case and once they get stuck in the cycle of sleep deprivation, it can quickly turn into more serious sleep troubles.

Insomnia can quickly develop in mothers who have the task of balancing taking care of the kids, sometimes work, keeping the house clean, running errands, and other obligations that no one else seems to be able to do. This constant jam-packed to-do list can only be accomplished when you sacrifice your time from somewhere else. For many mothers, the first thing they begin to cut back on in order to fit everything else in their day is their sleep.

Most moms will average around four hours of sleep for most of the first year of their baby's arrival, and after that, they will only get an additional hour of sleep until their baby turns two. The sleep deprivation does not end there either. Many moms will continue to run on little sleep until their child turns six, at which time additional activities and obligations begin to fill mom's schedule. The cycle just never seems to have an end in sight.

This is a severe problem for moms who want to be present and function on a daily basis. This long-term sleep deprivation can cause extreme irritability, fatigue, and lead to concentration problems. When you are always sleep deprived, you may eventually see issues with your vision, become increasingly lethargic, have poor eating habits, become disoriented frequently, have difficulty speaking clearly, or even be able to think clearly. Have you ever poured your baby's formula into your coffee cup and thought it was creamer or sugar? Chances are you are severely sleep-deprived. These minor mix-ups are often brushed off as not getting a good night's sleep, but consider how many more serious mix-ups you can have because you really are having too many interrupted sleep cycles. Hitting the gas pedal instead of the brake when driving? It happens all the time to sleep-deprived moms, and unfortunately, no one is taking these major mix-ups as a result of poor sleep.

Many moms are just told they are too stressed or anxious because of the baby's arrival and the new schedule and changes they are sorting through. But, more often than not, the stress, anxiety, and overwhelm moms feel is simply because they are not getting enough sleep. Losing sleep night after night can add to additional mental and physical health conditions that will only make sleeping more difficult. Postpartum depression, sleep apnea, and a range of anxiety disorders can be triggered just from becoming a mom but not getting the rest you need can also cause these conditions in new moms.

Sleep Apnea

Sleep apnea may have started while you were pregnant with your little and only magnifies once your baby has arrived. Sleep apnea occurs when there is an interruption to your breathing while you are sleeping. The airway tends to become blocked, which can cause:

- Excessive snoring
- Waking up feeling as though you have been choked
- Gasping for air in your sleep
- Sudden pausing in your breathing while asleep
- Increase in daytime drowsiness during the day

It is common for many women to suffer from sleep apnea while they are pregnant as their bodies change drastically to make room for their growing baby. But once the baby is born, sleep apnea can still affect and hinder your sleep, which only makes getting that quality sleep you desperately need even more difficult. On top of sleep apnea, many moms suffer from other forms of sleep disturbances that may linger after they have given birth:

- Restless leg syndrome
- Circadian rhythm sleep disorder
- Parasomnias
- Insomnia

These are common sleep disturbances in new moms. Many of these disorders are accepted as part of the role of being a new mom. When these conditions are left uncorrected, they intensify over the years. Even when your children are in school, a time when moms feel they will actually be able to get the rest they need, these sleep conditions can now prohibit you from a healthy sleep routine.

Postpartum Depression (PPD)

Sleep deprivation and postpartum depression have some similar side effects. Postpartum depression can have long-term effects on new moms that will often interfere with their abilities to care for their baby. The signs and symptoms are often subtle at first and overlooked as needing more time to adjust to having a new baby in the home. Sleep deprivation is closely linked to mom developing postpartum depression and will contribute to mom becoming affected by this type of depression for an extended period of time.

One of the biggest challenges for diagnosing postpartum depression is that it is common for many moms to go through a brief period of feeling the blues. Moms may find they cry over the simplest things or mistakes, will feel an increase in anxiety and have unpredictable mood swings. Often these postpartum symptoms will last for a few days or up to two weeks after having the baby. Postpartum depression, on the other hand, may show fewer signs at first but will have lingering symptoms after giving birth.

Signs of postpartum depression:

- Severe mood swings
- Depressed mood
- Detachment from baby; not feeling a bond or connection
- Withdrawing from family and friends
- Eating significantly less than usual
- Insomnia
- Lack of energy
- Fatigue
- Unable to find pleasure in activities once enjoyed

- Increase in anger or irritable
- Feelings of hopelessness
- Intense feelings of shame, guilt, and worthlessness
- Unable to think clearly or concentrate
- Being restless
- Panic attacks
- Thoughts of death or harm toward yourself or your baby

Mothers who suffer from postpartum depression often have difficulty getting quality sleep; even if they sleep for a full eight hours every night, they never feel as though they sleep well. This often is apparent in the mother's mood. When you are sleep deprived, it is understandable that you will feel more cranky and irritable; this usually goes away once you clock in those extra hours of sleep. Those with PPD, however, will have a serious change in their mood that can last for days and this can then cause mothers to become overly anxious and overwhelmed.

Postpartum depression can have an effect on many areas of your life. You may find you have no appetite, that you don't enjoy doing many things, or you lose the desire to participate in activities that once brought you joy. One of the biggest red flags of postpartum depression and the one that many mothers feel guilty for admitting is that they lack feeling a connection with their baby. Even mothers who are sleep deprived will have formed some sort of bond with their baby, but mothers who are suffering from PPD will notice they don't feel a connection with their little one. This lack of connection causes moms to fall even deeper into a depression as they begin to think they are not a good mom or are incapable of being a good mom to their baby.

Postpartum depression can last for months and even years after giving birth if untreated. For many moms, they do not even recognize the signs of this type of depression for months or even a year after having their baby.

Postpartum Psychosis (PPP)

Another less discussed condition that mothers may suffer from is known as postpartum psychosis. This is a serious condition that some mothers may experience within the first week have delivered their baby. Signs can include:

- Disorientation
- Confusion
- Hallucinations
- Delusion
- Obsessively thinking of your baby
- Sleep disturbances
- Increase in agitation
- Paranoia
- Excess energy
- May attempt to harm yourself or your baby

Though rare, this condition can be life-threatening to the mother or baby if not treated immediately. Those who have postpartum psychosis act in accordance to the delusion or hallucination they are perceiving. They can be completely unaware of the harm they are causing themselves or their child, as in their mind, these actions have been deemed as good or caring.

General Anxiety of a Young Mother

It is quite common for moms to feel a certain level of anxiety while they are pregnant and even after giving birth. Not only do you become more concerned about taking care of yourself, but you also become more concerned about staying healthy for your baby. You think that once your baby has arrived the anxiety will subdue for a short time, but you quickly find that a whole new set of worries come barreling over you. While it is normal for parents to worry about their child and it is not something you can ever expect to go away, there is a line between typical parental worries, such as is your child meeting their expected milestones, and those that cause you to irrationally feel concerned for the health and safety of your child.

Anxiety is an excessive form of worry that can be brought on for what seems to be no reason. You may find yourself wrapped up in fear when it comes to caring for your child so much so that you might fear taking them out of your home, even to go to doctor appointments. Many moms become afraid of having anxiety attacks when outside the home that they keep themselves locked up inside, day after day.

Anxiety is a natural response to fear, and a little anxiety can be healthy. Moms, however, tend to suffer through numerous anxiety attacks without ever realizing that their blood pressure is through the roof, their heart rate is erratic, and their mental clarity is completely distorted. So many moms get used to performing the same routines, day in and day out, they can run on autopilot without realizing that an anxiety attack is even occurring.

Postpartum Anxiety and Obsessive-Compulsive Disorder (PPA/OCD)

Postpartum anxiety and obsessive-compulsive disorder is often an overlooked concern that can affect mothers just as severely as postpartum depression. Those with postpartum anxiety/obsessive-compulsive disorder will find themselves submerged in traumatizing thoughts. These thoughts can revolve around:

- Their baby becoming a victim of Sudden Infant Death Syndrome
- Dropping their baby
- Finding their baby dead
- Baby choking
- The thought of shaking their baby
- Yelling at their baby
- Thought of their baby drowning while bathing them

Mothers who suffer from this form of OCD have a more difficult time resisting the urge to act out on their impulses, which can result in them choking their baby just to ensure they are, in fact, still alive. Many new moms have a fear of being left alone with their baby because of these intense impulses.

What should be noted: Just because you may have some of these unwanted thoughts that involve harm to your baby does not necessarily mean you have postpartum OCD. In fact, almost all new mothers have admitted that these thoughts have crept into their heads.

Solutions for You

No matter what, you always need to remember that taking care of yourself is just as important as taking care of your baby. If you do not take care of yourself, you will struggle when it comes to taking care of your baby. Also, keep in mind, your baby will often follow your sleep patterns even if you do not notice it. When mom is sleep-deprived and depressed, your baby will often have more difficulty sleeping. This spirals into a negative cycle where mom can't get enough sleep and becomes more depressed and baby doesn't sleep well, causing mom to sleep less and so on. To break the cycle of this negative sleep pattern, you need to take some necessary steps to ensure that you are getting quality sleep. Set up a sleep routine for yourself just as you have done for your child.

Some sleep routine suggestions:

- Create a relaxing sleep environment.
- Practice relaxation techniques such as deep breathing or meditation.
- Read.
- Journal.
- Prepare what you need before you lay down.
- Soak in warm water with lavender oil or bath salts (be careful not to fall asleep while bathing).
- Invest in a quality mattress, blankets, pillows, and sleepwear. The more comfortable you are, the easier it will be to drift to sleep.

While worrying about your child is a normal part of parenting, these worries can develop into more serious concerns. Mothers who have postpartum depression, postpartum anxiety, or obsessive-compulsive disorder are more likely to cause harm to their baby or themselves. Sleep is a key factor when it comes to developing these issues.

Do not be afraid or embarrassed to ask for help or to have a trusted family member come take over for you so you can get the sleep you need. If at any point you may be concerned about your mood, behavior, or sleep struggles, reach out to your doctor. You may benefit from talking with a therapist who can provide you with additional tools that will allow you to de-stress and worry less so that you can sleep and be a better mom for your child.

Key Points to Remember

- Just as you expect your little one to stick with their sleep routine, you need to implement those rules for yourself as well. You, your baby, and the rest of the household will all benefit from it.
- Sleep disorders are common with moms, but that doesn't mean you have to suffer from them.
- Never hesitate to talk to your doctor if you are struggling with sleep yourself.
- Ask for help. Raising a baby is hard; no one will look down or think less of you.

CHAPTER 11: Personal Note – Mom to Mom

As a mother myself, I completely understand all the emotions you are feeling. I understand the thoughts of "Did I do my best?" and "What could I have done differently?" that you have coursing through your mind every day. I understand the stress and the struggles that you have internally—the ones that no one sees, but you know they are there because you feel them. You may feel them stronger one moment and less the next moment. Sometimes, they make you feel that you are going crazy.

But let me tell you something that I know you do not hear enough—*You are amazing and you are doing your best!* You need to take a moment (or more) every day to note how well you are doing as a mother and feel proud of yourself. I know how hard this is because we often look to other people to lift our spirits, but sometimes we need to do it ourselves. In fact, it is healthy to make sure that you take time to tell yourself the following statements every day:

- No matter how chaotic today was, I did my best and I am proud of myself for doing so.
- I am a great mother because I am doing my best.
- It is okay to make mistakes. They happen and this allows me to grow as a parent.
- I did what I could today. Just because there are dirty dishes in the sink and the laundry is piled up does not mean I did not do my best. I took care of myself and my baby. These are my priorities.
- My baby does not expect me to be perfect, so I do not expect

myself to do perfectly.
- The time I spent with my baby today was not a waste. Their time means more to me than any chores or errands I could have done.
- I am the best person to raise my baby.
- Everyone raises their baby differently. If someone does not like the way I raise my baby, that is fine. I am doing what is best for my baby and this is what matters.

I remember needing to repeat the last point to myself the most throughout the day. It seems that no matter what we share on Facebook, Twitter, Instagram, or any other social media site (or even with people face-to-face), there are always critics. There is always that parent who would "do it this way" or "do it better." There are always people who are not even parents that have an idea of how to raise your child. You might have the in-laws who do not believe you are raising your baby right. Whoever the person is, you always need to remember that they are giving their opinions. Respect their opinions and continue to do what you are doing because no matter what anyone else says, you are their parent. You are your child's parent, you are their nurturer, you know what is right for them. The only person who should make decisions along with you when it comes to raising your baby is the baby's other parent, whether you are co-parenting or married.

The best statement to remember when it comes to criticism or other parents telling you what you should do is follow your instincts. *You are the best person to raise your child and no one knows them better than you.*

Oh, patience. How it wears thin often when you are a parent, even to a baby. Patience is one of the main keys when it comes to sleep training and it is hard to always have patience. There will be times when you lack patience, you feel irritated, you just want your baby to sleep, and you might be in tears begging God to help you. When it comes down to these moments, take a step back and take some time to yourself. I promise, if you walk out of your baby's room for a couple of minutes to regain your composure and find more patience, nothing bad will happen to your baby. In fact, you can walk back into the room and find that your baby is calmer because you are calmer. Always remember that your baby feeds off of how you feel and this will affect how they act.

Do not feel guilty by walking out of the room. You need to take care of yourself and this means more than just making sure you get the sleep you need during the night. You need to take care of yourself emotionally, physically, and mentally. You need to be gentle with yourself. Think of it this way—if you would not talk a certain way to someone else, why would you talk that way to yourself? Yes, you are your worst critic when it comes to being a mom, but the more your practice gentleness with yourself, the more you can teach your child to be gentle with other people.

Now, I will share with you the words of wisdom my mother told me: *This too shall pass.* At the time I did not want to hear it, as some of you now might not be interested in hearing those four words. But, this phrase is true. Every part of your child's life will pass. The struggle with sleep training will pass. The struggle with sleep regression will pass. Soon, your child will start talking, crawling, walking, and running, and you will wonder where the time has gone. You will have moments when you miss them at this age and wish you could shrink them back to that size, just to hold them a little longer. Believe me, this does happen.

Remember, you are not alone. You are not the only mother going through the difficulties of sleep training. You are not the only mother who is listening to their baby crying as you try to calm them by caressing their cheek. There are thousands of other mothers who know exactly what you are going through and they are willing to lend a helping hand. One of the best steps I took when I started sleep training was joining a couple of Facebook groups. I met several mothers who offered their advice and, more importantly, support. Sometimes it is the support that will give you the extra patience or the strength you need to carry on with sleep training when you do not think you are succeeding. They also give you support when it comes to being a mother. Of course, there are many who will criticize you, but I started to focus more on the mothers who tried to help as they were the reasons why I was there.

Out of everything we discussed in this book, the most significant piece of information I want you to take with you is that parenthood is an amazing and fulfilling adventure. You will have one struggle after the next, but they all will pass. You are teaching your child every step of the way, even when you do not feel they are listening (if you have not gotten to this point yet with any of your children, you will). You are doing great because you are doing your best. As stated before, your child does not need a perfect parent, they need *you. You are amazing.*

Now I want you to repeat that to yourself. *I am amazing.*

CONCLUSION

No matter where you are in your sleep training journey, you know that your baby needs to feel safe and loved. You are doing everything in your power to do this and you are doing an excellent job. You are an amazing mom and you need to be proud of your journey.

Raising a child is a difficult task but also one of the most rewarding. Once you have overcome the sleep obstacles so that you and your baby are well-rested, you will be able to enjoy the precious moments you share with one another. You should feel relieved that there is hope and a solution for all those restless nights and frustrations you have encountered up until now.

There is a lot of information that you learned in this book and it can start to feel a little overwhelming at times, especially if you are a first-time mom. Through these pages, you have gained a clear understanding of how vital it is for you and your baby to get the right amount of sleep. Not only do you now have the knowledge to ensure your baby is sleeping enough, you also have a number of tools to help you implement an effective sleep routine.

Sleeping training from an early age allows your baby to learn and adjust to the many changes they will be confronted with as they grow. You are providing your child with the skills and tools they can utilize for the rest of their life to continue to develop healthy sleep patterns. Rest assured, though you may be challenged at first, the benefits far exceed the temporary struggles.

This book has clearly outlined how to determine the amount of sleep your baby needs based on their age and points out the key factors that can cause their sleep disturbances during these times. You now know when to expect sleep regression and how to create an action plan that will ensure your baby falls back into a healthy sleep routine. You have an effective step-by-step plan that guides your baby to self-sooth with minimal tears and fears.

This book has given you priceless information that will benefit your baby as well as you, their mom. Remember that your sleep is just as important as theirs. The best piece of advice I can give you is to take it one moment at a time. No, not one day at a time—one moment at a time. There are a lot of moments that are wrapped up in one day and your emotions will fly everywhere. Therefore, it is best to go moment by moment as this will help ease your stress and keep you calm.

BONUS SECTION: Guided Meditation for Parents - Putting Your Baby to Sleep

In this bonus section, I have prepared a special one and a half hours guided meditation session for you, the parent, to be able to cope with the sleep training journey in the most positive and relaxed way. The best time to listen to this meditation would be just before putting your baby to sleep, just relax and dive in. I know that as a sleep deprived parent you do not have an hour to spare - simply listen to this right after you have put your baby in their crib and while you are following the step you are at in this process.

If this is the audio version, just dive in.
If this is the kindle or paperback version, sit down and read it to yourself slowly.

-Over the next few moments, you will emerge in a complete state of focus and calmness. Listening to this guided meditation will slowly begin to feel natural, easy and relaxing. You will completely relax just by listening to this recording and the sound of my voice and the sounds around it.

-Begin by focusing on your breath. Notice the breath gently, as the air goes into your lungs and then comes back out again.

-Breath normally, but notice the movement of the chest expanding as you inhale, and then reducing as you exhale the air out of your body.

-Feel the stream of air going in, staying there for a moment, and then coming out again.

-Gently, prepare to enter a world of calm, of clarity and comfort as you prepare to tuck your baby to sleep. Prepare for the rewarding practice of teaching them sleep, the essential part of human life that lets us rest and come back to life every morning.

-Imagine being on a beautiful beach covered with serene, golden sand from one end to the other. The water is calm, the small waves crashing into the fine shore. The sun is just about to set while the breeze of the sea touches every pore on your skin.

-Breathe in, feeling the fresh breezy air expanding your lungs, and then breathe out, letting all of the stress and worry of the day flow into the atmosphere with your exhalation.

-You are doing wonderfully.

-After this next breath, continue to relax as you begin to do a short checkup on the entire body.

-Breathing out, focus on the top of your head. See how it feels up there, just gently checking if it is warm, cold, if it is still or fuzzy. Don't try to change anything, but simply notice the feelings, and then move along.

-Continue going down to the face. See just how your face is feeling right now, without judgement. See if it feels tense or relaxed, notice if it is straight or with a grimase. However it is, simply notice it, don't try to change it and then move along.

-Next, feel the back of the head. Get a sense of how it feels back there, if it is clear or fuzzy, cold or a tad warm, if you can feel any tension or not at all.

-Whatever it is that you feel, you only notice the sensation and let go without trying to change anything. Breathe slowly as you do so, gently, and notice as your breath becomes softer and calmer with each body part that you're checking on.

-Move down to the neck, the place where the spine meets the head. Gently feel the sensations and warmth of the neck. Notice how it stands, if it's straight or on one side or the other, without the need to change anything. Breathe in, and then breathe out feeling the air passing through it.

-You are doing wonderfully. Breathe in, focusing on your neck, then breathe out, letting go of all anguish, stress, anger, unpleasantness, tension.

-It is now time to focus on the chest area and the upper back. Begin by scanning your chest. Is your chest tough or relaxed today? Is it tense or calm? Feel the beating heart in the middle of it, the source of your life. Try to feel the flow of blood through the main vessels of your chest, pumping throughout your entire body.

-Move your attention to the upper back. How is this part of the body right now? Regardless if it feels well or unwell, simply notice it and then continue to breathe calmly, as evenly and normally as possible. Relax your shoulders, your chest and your upper back.

-You are now scanning down your stomach and lower back. Begin by feeling the sensations in your stomach. Is your stomach full or empty right now? Is it bloated, or flat? Whatever the case, simply notice the feelings in the stomach while breathing in, and then breathing out gently.

-Focus on the lower back now. Gently scan the middle of your back and then move down the spine to the base of it. Feel it for how it is right at this moment, without judgement or uneasiness from your part. Notice the sensations in the lower back as you first breathe in, and then gently release the air out.

-You are doing just wonderfully.

-Next it is time to focus your attention on the upper part of your legs. Notice any sensations of tingling, relaxation, tension or calm in the legs. Moving down, focus on your knee caps and back of the knees. Look for any sensations that might feel natural or different. Then, move along to the bottom part of your legs, gently searching for any sensations.

-Whatever these sensations might be, all you have to do is notice them in a calm, unbiased manner. You don't have to interfere with them, you don't have to get angry at them, all you have to do is simply notice them, and then move on as you breathe in and out.

-You have now arrived at the feet. Start noticing what sort of sensations you can feel from the back of the feet all the way to the toes. Is there any tingling, or tension, or are the feet gentle, relaxed? Breathe in, feeling the feet relaxing without moving them, and then breathe out, letting the entire body relax.

-At last, feel the sensations that are now present in your arms. Starting with the upper arms, moving down to the elbows, and then all the way to the hands and fingers. See if you can distinguish any sensations, any tensions or calmness. And as you do so, breathing in and out in a natural manner, let go of any tension you can feel anywhere in the body.

-Before moving forward with this meditation, take a moment to appreciate the moment of now.

-Remember to just breathe gently as you appreciate this sense of calm, of stillness throughout the body as you prepare to put your child to rest. Do it in a gentle, motherly way only you can, showing your kid the love and appreciation he or she deserves.

-And as you do so, start imagining a bolt of white light coming from the ceiling right above your head. The light is warm to the touch as it reaches the top of your head, gently warming your hair and skin. The light keeps flowing from somewhere up all the way to your head, and as it reaches the neck the entire head feels lighter, less tense and still.

-The beam of light now moves to the area where the chest is. When it reaches the chest, you will immediately feel a sense of lightness, of easiness and space in the chest. Any ache, trouble or discomfort will dissipate as the light spreads through every bone, every muscle, every cavity of the heart in the middle of your body.

-Just like that, you will now breathe in, and then breathe out.

-The light now reaches the stomach area of the body. If this area felt tense or uneasy a moment ago, the moment the beam of light reaches the stomach, it becomes still, untroubled. The sense of calm and clarity overflows in the middle of your body, creating a sense of space and positivity.

-The beam of light is now making its way to the top of your legs and the knees. As it reaches this part of the body, you start to feel even more relaxed, even more aware of everything that happens inside or outside of the body.

-The light calms any tension down from your legs and knees, which are responsible with the noble task of carrying you around every single day. It warms the legs up and makes them stronger and more efficient.

-As the light travels down to the feet, the entire body is enveloped in a sense of stillness like you've never felt before. There is no tension, no stress, no bothering, just you and the beam of light that has now reached every single muscle, bone, tissue, piece of skin, even cell in your body.

-The light creates a sense of space between you the material, and you the spiritual. You can feel the space as you'd hit the pause button on a music player. Every time you visualise the beam of light coming down over you, you'll be able to hit the pause button and create that space.

-And every time you'll do so, you will feel relaxed, stress-free and lighter.

-Remember to visualise the beam of light whenever you need to, as doing so will increase the powerful, beneficial effects it can have on the body and mind. The more you practice this part of the meditation regardless of your situation, the better it will be for you, and also for the people around you.

-It is now time to come back to the senses in your body and out. Begin by taking a big breath, breathing in through the nose, and then out through the mouth. And as you do so, start to use the five senses in order to bring yourself back to the moment.

-Begin by using the sense of sound in your ears. See if you can distinguish any sounds, those that are particularly close to you, like birds singing outside the window, a washing machine working somewhere in the background, or even people chatting on the street.

-Continue by distinguishing those sounds that are further from you. Try to hear some cars passing by on a road that's further from your home, any louder sounds that might come from a factory, or even a jet plane passing way above your head.

-As you refine and activate your sense of sound, remember to be thankful for having it and for it working for you every single day. Become more aware of the sense of sound, as you become more aware of the air and space around you.

-You are now going to focus on your sense of touch and general feeling of the body. This sense is available all over your body, anywhere that there's skin. Start by feeling the air on your face and hands and feet, if your legs or arms are not totally covered.

-Now focus on the areas of the body that can sense clothes. Try to feel the fibers the clothes are made out of. Pass the sensation of just skin touching the clothing and focus on the materials that are enhancing your capabilities to feel things. Remember to feel with your entire body, starting with the head, neck, chest and back, stomach area, moving down to the upper legs, knees, lower legs, feet and hands.

--As you refine and activate your sense of feeling, remember to be grateful for having it and for it working for you every single day. Become more aware of the sense of touch, as you become more aware of the space and air around you.

-It is now time to get even more in contact with the present moment by activating your sense of smell. Try smelling the entire room you and your child are in. What is the most pungent smell anywhere in the room? Simply notice it and feel it going down your olfactory canals without judgement.

-Now, move into the sense of smell a little deeper. Distinguish a few smells that aren't that pungent but are still present in the room. They can be smells of toys, of foods, even the smell of your baby, which is so important to any parent. Recognise the smells and observe them, as you enhance your overall sense of presence.

-As you activate and refine your sense of smell, remember to be thankful for having it and for it working for you every single day. Become more aware of the sense of smell, as you become more aware of the air and space around you.

-Breathe in, and then breathe out gently. You are doing wonderfully.

-The time has come now to focus on your fourth sense, which is the sense of taste. You don't have to bite into something to reactivate this sense. Simply open your mouth and see which tastes activate in your mouth. It could be a floral taste, or something that has to do with your previous meal.

-Whatever it might be, simply notice the sensation of taste on your tongue and everywhere in your mouth without trying to change anything about it. Tasting is so important for you as a parent, as it enables you to taste the food of your kid and make sure it is just right.

-And as you refine and once again activate your sense of taste, remember to be grateful for having it and for it working for you every single day. Become more aware of the sense of taste, as you become more aware of the space and air around you.

-The final sense you'll be reactivating during this part of the meditation is the sense of sight. Seeing the things around you will happen slowly, gradually. Begin by closing and then gently opening your eyes, like you'd come out of a nap.

-Start by visualising the very first, largest object in your sight. It might be a mirror, a television, or a dresser. Whatever it might be, try to focus your sight on the shape of the object without regarding what it actually is. Look for its colour, shape, size, but don't emphasise on the actual thing that it is. Look for the small details of this object and see them for what they are.

-Next, move along the sight and see what other objects are in the room. Focus on their shapes, sizes and colors, without mentally naming them or judging them in any way. Simply see them for what they are, shapes and sizes and colors that form objects.

-Finally, as you refine and once again activate your sense of sight, remember to be grateful for having it and for it working for you every single day. Become more aware of the sense of sight, as you become more aware of the space and air around you.

-You are doing great. Breathe in and then breathe out slowly. Feel the expansion and then the contraction of the chest and how every single cell in your body is filled with life as the air moves around the entire body.

-We are now going to be focusing on the breath, the essential process of life on Earth. Breathing is what keeps humans, animals and plants alive. Oxygen is coming in through our noses, feeding the lungs and the entire body, and then carbon monoxide is released into the atmosphere. The plants are breathing in what we breathe out, while we breathe in what the plants are exhaling, forming the complete circle of life as we know it.

-Exploring the breath, begin by taking a few big, deep breaths in through the nose, and out through the mouth.

-And as we will explore the breath in the next couple of minutes, remember to find the time and space to prepare for your child going to sleep. Being close to them, notice how he or she sits, behaves and looks. Put away any judgement, stress or tension in your observation. Simply observe the beautiful human being next to you, cherishing the present time you have together.

-And as you exhale one last time, close your eyes and give your breath a few seconds to get back to a steady, normal rate.

-Breathe in through the nose, and then again out through the nose, like you'd normally do.

-And as you do so, begin to observe the airways that start from the tip of your nose and go straight into the lungs where the breathing happens. Start focusing on the very top of the nose, right underneath the tip of it, where the air first meets the body while you inhale.

-Create a soft, gentle focus on that very spot. For a few moments now, focus on nothing but that place of contact between the air and the beginning of the nose. Completely focus your attention on that spot alone, as you inhale, and then exhale.

-You are doing a great job. Keep focusing, applying a gentle, pure focus on the spot.

-Next, while continuing to focus on the tip of the nose when inhaling and exhaling, we'll move a little closer to the source of breathing, which is the air. Divide your attention between that first place of contact, and the air that goes into your lungs and then back out.

-As soon as you breathe in, focus your attention on the stream of air cooling down your body. Feel as the air travels from the nose to the lungs through the larynx, trachea, bronchi and then into the lungs.

-While the air is there, sitting for just a few seconds, appreciate the entire capacity of breathing, the thing that makes us a living being. Become conscious of how the breath forms from outside the body, then inside and then out once more.

-Become more conscious of the breathing in and breathing out process of breathing.

-Before you let the air move out of the lungs again, focus your attention on the warm air that you are breathing out of your body. How it moves from the lungs up through the bronchi, trachea and larynx, reaching the nose and then moving out.

-At the end of the exhale, once again, shift your focus to the area just below the tip of your nose, where the last contact with air is being made as you exhale, applying a gentle focus on that spot at all times.

-While your eyes are still closed, you are going to spend a few moments repeating this process by yourself. Gently feel the air at the tip of the nose as it goes in, moves down to the lungs in a cold airstream, sits there for a moment, then moves back up in a warm stream and then touches the tip of the nose once more before leaving the body.

-Great, you are doing perfectly.

-And now slowly get back to the body and the physical world around you. Start by feeling the touch of your body on the chair or the bed where you sit.

-Continue by feeling the sensations in the body, see if the body is warm or a little colder, if it is tense or relaxed, if it feels comfortable or uncomfortable.

-Get back to the moment of now by activating the sense of sound, listening to those sounds that are closer to you, and then to those that are a little further as well. See if you can listen to the sound of a bird singing, an airplane passing by or just a car driving away in the distance.

-And as you do so, open your eyes gently and use the sense of sight to fully become aware of the space around you. See the room you're in, the child that's beside you and the connection between the two of you.

-You will now begin to focus on the primal connection between you and the child that you love so dearly. Begin by observing your child without making any mental notes about it. Simply use the senses to consciously feel the presence of your child near you.

-This life that you've created is the most important thing for you in the entire Universe. It is the only person you can love unconditionally the most out of all. It is the essence of your entire life, both physical and mental.

-As you continue to observe this child that you brought into this life, take a moment to appreciate the importance of rest and sleep in your life, as well as your child's life. Imagine feeling fresh, rested and ready to go after a long, satisfying sleep.

-Your child needs sleep as much as you do, which is why understanding the importance of teaching your child to sleep independently, is key for a smoother, more enjoyable process.

-Sleep helps your child to grow better, to become a healthier being and to understand the world around them much deeper. At his or her age, your child knows absolutely nothing about the importance of sleep. This is why you might feel like they are trying their best to not fall asleep.

-They in fact simply don't know better, which is why putting them to sleep might seem like a tedious process. The process is natural, it happens not only with humans but with all life on Earth in the same way.

-As the parent of this child, while continuing to gently focus on your breathing and becoming more and more aware about the importance of sleep, you will help your child soothe themselves to sleep in a gentle, loving manner.

-From now on, every time your child feels like they are resisting falling asleep, you will know better and gently, softly help them. You will become more relaxed, more ready and more patient with their resistance, knowing it is a natural response of a being that does not know the importance of sleep yet.

-From now on, every time your child will cry when put to bed, you will patiently wait for them to relax, comforting them with the warmth of your hands, and if needed your body, the place where they will feel at ease and safer than anywhere else.

-From now on, as soon as your child relaxes and gets ready to sleep, regardless of how much time it took him or her, you will not judge them for anything and not regard the experience as being a tedious one, but a normal, natural and loving one.

-You are doing just great. Remember to breathe in through the nose, and then again out through the nose as you'd normally do. Simply focusing on the breath gently, without forcing anything. Just remembering there's the breath for you to come back to over and over again, whenever things feel tight or uneasy.

-We are now approaching the end of this meditation session. Take a few moments to appreciate the calming sensation of ease and relaxation surrounding you.

-Appreciate the warmth of the connection between you and your child. See it for what it truly represents: a primordial link that's unbreakable by anybody or anything on this planet.

-Be grateful for being able to have such a valuable connection that no material gains can compare to. Appreciate the feelings of pure love you send to and receive from this wonderful being.

-Completely relax now as you take a deep breath in through the nose, and then out through the mouth.

-One last time now, gently close your eyes as you breathe in and out through the nose.

-Remembering the sensation of the beam of light from a little later, imagine a beam of light over your head again, this time filling your body from the tips of your toes to the top of your head with relaxation and calmness. This time, as soon as you visualise the light coming down and filling your body, the sensation appears almost instantly.

-Sit for a few seconds and appreciate the sensations of calm, space and bliss. Make a pact with yourself to keep this sensation with you throughout the day and night, while caring for your child and putting them to bed, feeding them or simply being there for them. Keep yourself this way every second of every day. And when you feel like things are rough, simply return to the breath and the beam of light that cures the body and the mind of all tensions.

-Once again, breathe in through the nose and then one final time out through the nose.

-Gently open your eyes, and appreciate the feeling of relaxation that enveloped your entire being. Your meditation session has now completed.

RESOURCES

12-Month Sleep Regression. (2019, August 10). Retrieved from https://www.tuck.com/12-month-sleep-regression/

A bedtime routine to put your baby to sleep. (n.d). Retrieved from https://www.nestedbean.com/blogs/zen-blog/bedtime-routine

American Academy of Pediatrics Announces New Safe Sleep Recommendations to Protect Against SIDS, Sleep-Related Infant Deaths. (2016, October 24). Retrieved from https://www.aap.org/en-us/about-the-aap/aap-press-room/Pages/American-Academy-of-Pediatrics-Announces-New-Safe-Sleep-Recommendations-to-Protect-Against-SIDS.aspx

Brown, C. (2017, June 14). Surviving the 8-10 month sleep regression. Retrieved from https://bellalunasleep.com/surviving-8-10-month-sleep-regression/

Bruise, C. (2019, November 6). How to handle your toddler's 18-month sleep regression. Retrieved from https://www.verywellfamily.com/your-toddler-s-18-month-sleep-regression-4159537

Co-sleeping with your baby: advice from The Lullaby Trust. (n.d.). Retrieved from https://www.lullabytrust.org.uk/safer-sleep-advice/co-sleeping/

Decoding Your Baby's 7 Types of Cries (2019, April 15). Retrieved from https://www.whattoexpect.com/first-year/week-10/decoding-cries.aspx

Ding, K. (n.d). Can I train my baby to fall asleep without leaving him to cry? Retrieved from https://www.babycenter.com/0_baby-sleep-training-no-tears-methods_1497581.bc

Dubinsky, D. (n.d.). What is the cry it out method? Retrieved from https://www.babycenter.com/0_baby-sleep-training-cry-it-out-methods_1497112.bc

Ednick, M., Cohen, A. P., McPhail, G. L., Beebe, D., Simakajornboon, N., & Amin, R. S. (2009, November). A review of the effects of sleep during the first year of life on cognitive, psychomotor, and temperament development. Sleep. Retrieved from https://www.ncbi.nlm.nih.gov/pmc/articles/PMC2768951/

Establishing good sleep habits: newborn to three months. (2017, January). Retrieved from https://www.babycentre.co.uk/a7654/establishing-good-sleep-habits-newborn-to-three-months

How to establish a good baby sleep routine. (n.d.). Retrieved from https://www.aptaclub.co.uk/baby/health-and-wellbeing/stress-and-sleep/how-to-establish-good-baby-sleep-routine.html

How to reduce the risk of SIDS for your baby. (n.d.). Retrieved from https://www.lullabytrust.org.uk/safer-sleep-advice/

Infant Sleep. (n.d.). What Are the sleep Needs of an Infant? Retrieved from http://www.columbianeurology.org/neurology/staywell/document.php?id=36578

Moon, R. (2019, April 15). How to Keep Your Sleeping Baby Safe: AAP Policy Explained. Retrieved from https://www.healthychildren.org/English/ages-stages/baby/sleep/Pages/A-Parents-Guide-to-Safe-Sleep.aspx

Newborn sleep routines. (2018, May 6). Retrieved from https://raisingchildren.net.au/newborns/sleep/settling-routines/newborn-sleep-routines

Reduce the risk of sudden infant death syndrome (SIDS). (2018, September 17). Retrieved from https://www.nhs.uk/conditions/pregnancy-and-baby/reducing-risk-cot-death/

Schiedel, B. (2019, May 2). Sleep and feeding schedules for your baby and toddler. Retrieved from https://www.todaysparent.com/baby/baby-sleep/sleep-and-feeding-schedules-for-your-baby-and-toddler/

STTN: What does Sleeping Through the Night Really Mean? (2017, December 14). Retrieved from https://www.munchkin.com/blog/sleeping-through-the-night/

Your Baby and the Fourth Trimester. (n.d). Retrieved from https://www.babycentre.co.uk/a25019365/your-baby-and-the-fourth-trimester

Your Guide to Managing the 4-Month Sleep Regression. (2016, February 5). Retrieved from https://www.healthline.com/health/parenting/4-month-sleep-regression#The-Takeaway

Weissbluth, M. (2005). *Healthy Sleep Habits, Happy Child. A Step-by-Step Program for Good Night's Sleep.* New York, NY: Ballantine Books

Manufactured by Amazon.ca
Bolton, ON